CONTROVERSIES IN HEALTH CARE POLICIES:
POLICIES:
CHALLENGES TO PRACTICE

CONTROVERSIES IN HEALTH CARE POLICIES: CHALLENGES TO PRACTICE

Edited by
Marshall Marinker
*Director of Medical Education, MSD Ltd,
and Visiting Professor of General Practice,
UMDS, London*

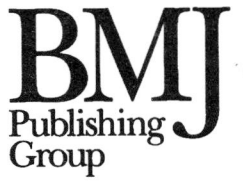

BMJ
Publishing
Group

© BMJ Publishing Group 1994

First published in 1994
Reprinted 1995
Reprinted September 1995
by the BMJ Publishing Group, BMA House, Tavistock Square,
London WC1H 9JR

British Library Cataloguing in Publication Data

A catalogue record for this book is available
from the British Library

ISBN 0-7279-0894-4

Printed and bound in Great Britain by
Latimer Trend & Company Ltd., Plymouth

Contents

About the partner organisation

Social Market Foundation

The Social Market Foundation is a registered charity and a company limited by guarantee. Since it was established in 1989, it has become one of Britain's most influential think tanks. It is frequently consulted by senior ministers and officials and its meetings bring together cabinet ministers, staff from 10 Downing Street, opposition politicians, academics and thinkers, senior journalists, and practitioners in the business world.

Through its programme of publications, seminars, and conferences, the foundation has helped shape the political and economic debate. Its research into issues such as the reform of the public sector and the conduct of economic policy has found an audience across the political spectrum.

King's fund

The King's Fund seeks to stimulate good practice and innovation in all aspects of health care and management through service developments, education, policy analysis, audit, and direct grants.

Health care services in London and the health of Londoners remain its primary concern. The fund also supports work further afield if that provides a relevant model for London. It always tries to set its work in a national and international context.

Working closely with health authorities and hospitals, the fund uses its income to: make grants to improve health care, improve management in health services, encourage innovation and the adoption of good practice in health care, clarify health policy, and publish reports of projects and studies supported by the Fund.

National Association of Health Authorities and Trusts

The National Association of Health Authorities and Trusts (NAHAT) is the association for NHS boards and the voice of the NHS management family. It brings together all sectors of the health service – family health services authorities, health authorities, GP fundholders, and NHS trusts. And importantly, it provides an effective forum through which they are able to exchange their views and ideas.

Age Concern

As the National Council on Ageing, Age Concern England pursues its goals through the development of services for older people, the provision of information and advice, publications, grants, training of voluntary and professional carers, and campaigning, fundraising, and marketing. It works closely with partner organisations in the UK, Europe and internationally, and is committed to teaching and research.

Royal College of General Practitioners

The Royal College of General Practitioners was founded in 1952, with this object:

"To encourage, foster, and maintain the highest possible standards in general practice and for that purpose to take or join with others in taking steps consistent with the charitable nature of that object which may assist towards the same."

Medical Advisers Support Centre

The Medical Advisers Support Centre (MASC) was set up by the Department of Health in 1990 and acts as an information and resource centre for family health services authority (FHSA) advisers.

Medical and pharmaceutical advisers are appointed by the FHSAs to provide advice to general practitioners and FHSAs on "improving prescribing" and on other issues relating to primary health care.

MASC offers support and training for professional advisers in four major areas: therapeutics and clinical pharmacology, general topics related to prescribing, management skills, and individual skills.

Preface

In 1994 MSD Ltd initiated a programme of medical education workshops and health care policy think tanks, papers, and seminars, designed to address some of the challenges of a rapidly changing health service. In pursuit of this, six important health care topics were identified. These were not the subject of intense and public debate and conflict, but appeared to be important and interesting parts of the infrastructure of health care thinking on which so much policy making must rest.

In relation to each of these topics it was possible to secure the partnership of a major national organisation. *Age Concern* became a partner in looking at the implications of the boundary between ageing and disease; *King's Fund* in looking at risk in medicine; *National Association of Health Authorities and Trusts* in the problems inherent in medical practice variation; *Medical Advisers Support Centre* in how we judge improvements in primary health care; *Royal College of General Practitioners* in rational prescribing, and *Social Market Foundation* in looking at what sort of information about health and health care ought to be made available to the public.

Each of these organisations gave enthusiastic support to the relevant think tank, and I am grateful to all the members of our groups who gave so generously of their time and expertise. Our meetings were lively, and the contributions often controversial, surprising, and innovative. Much of this has been captured by our authors, whose fortitude and forbearance during many redrafts eased the job of the editor. I want also to record my particular thanks to Deborah Reece of BMJ Books, for constant help and wise counsel.

We offer this collection of essays as a contribution to what we hope will become a much broader debate, beyond specialist circles, of the hard choices which constitute public policy about health care.

Marshall Marinker
October 1994

Chapter 1
Evidence, paradox, and consensus

Marshall Marinker

Introduction

In choosing the six topics that form the basis of this collection of essays, one of my expectations was that we would avoid major areas of public controversy concerning the current NHS reforms. Instead we would look at some of the underlying issues—the nature of risk in medicine; entitlement to access by the public to information about medicine, health, and the health service; the large variations in medical practice and what this implies for policy; the meaning of aging and its relation to our ideas about health, disease and treatment; the sort of criteria that we should be applying to judgments about quality in primary health care; a rational approach to prescribing. None of these issues, in themselves, was self evidently the stuff of political dispute.

Each of the topics was tackled by a group of experts and enthusiasts. They were discussed over two or three one-day meetings, during which a variety of views was expressed, experiences shared, and differences explored. The groups or think tanks were not making policy. They were exploring some of the infrastructures of policy making. What ensued was a lively dialogue, which contributed to each writer's final reports (the subsequent chapters in this book). The members of the group, therefore, may have influenced but did not seek to determine the content, style, or moral tone of what was eventually written. Although the members of the groups were not making policy, something of the process of policy making was being enacted.

As convenor of all six groups I was privileged to be their only common member. As a result of this experience three salient features of policy making in health care impressed themselves on me:

- The profound uncertainities and ambiguities in medicine that masquerade as facts
- The pervasiveness of conflicting ideas and values
- The complexity of the group process by which we come to an agreement about what to do.

These three factors, the nature of evidence, paradox, and consensus, are explored further in this opening chaper which arrives at an all too predictable conclusion. This is the importance of moving from polemic to dialogue if we are to arrive at health care policies that will be relatively safe, relatively relevant, and relatively acceptable to the public in whose name they are created and carried out.

Evidence

Whatever the political philosophies and professional or other self interests which divide party politicians, health care workers, patients, and so on, the assumptions on which debate turns, the tools of rhetoric employed, are remarkably similar. These concern the primacy of the "facts" on which all logical argument purports to be founded. There is a declared respect for evidence—about needs, about outcomes, about risk, about cost, and about benefit. Of course there will be preferences about which pieces of evidence to quote, and about how to interpret them. But "facts are facts." Yet often, when we come to examine evidence, the so-called facts about medicine and health care appear to be less scientifically factual, than morally factitious. I shall argue that health care policy, like clinical practice, is conditioned by the inherent uncertainties which characterise the biological and social sciences from which we derive most of our descriptions of health and disease. The theme of uncertainty recurred throughout the six sets of discourse.

Hills[1] in a *British Medical Journal* leader reiterates an often repeated anxiety that our education system, perhaps even our lives, is crammed too full of facts. Although he uses the word "knowledge" throughout his piece, he is quite clearly referring to facts. He writes: "Our preoccupation with knowledge has led to a serious neglect of other forms of learning . . . And yet skills, especially intellectual skills, are the very stuff of life, of jobs, and certainly of wealth creation." He concludes: "knowledge is luggage, and it would be best to travel light."

Randomised controlled trials (RCTs) represent perhaps the gold standard of facts about medical treatment. They are often large scale, can be aggregated for the purposes of meta-analysis, and are costly in resources and time. Although they may provide the best evidence available on the outcome of alternative strategies, they cannot themselves predict the individual choices which the clinician will make about his patients, or the policy maker about some development of the service.

Medical practice variations

In chapter 4 on medical practice variations it is noted that variations arose not only because doctors and others ignored the best evidence from RCTs but also because of the inherent uncertainties about so much in medical care. The variation in hysterectomy rates, for example, strongly suggest that gynaecologists have no sound criteria for either diagnosis or treatment of the symptoms that lead to the surgery. Variations in GPs' prescribing throw similar doubts on the solidity of agreed criteria for much diagnosis and treatment in primary care. Yet such is the hunger for the "facts", that rational prescribing is most often expressed as the achievement of mean values, as though there were some evident democratic virtue in the average of irrational behaviours.

Most of the facts that we have about medicine—the description of diseases, their natural history, the likely outcome of treatments—are the expressions of averages within groups. We may say of a particular patient that the evidence suggests that, given his age and condition, the results of treatment are likely to be only minimal relief from symptoms over a relatively short period of time. This may be misleading, however, even though the best evidence is being adduced. The minimal improvement in symptoms, the short time span, are simply averages, and the averages conceal the range of the findings from which they are calculated. Who is to say that this particular patient will not obtain considerable relief of symptoms over many years? Only the exercise of clinical judgment, a consideration of both the context and the content of the patient's problem, can inform the necessary choices. To dismiss the role of judgment, including the use of implicit knowledge and intuitive thinking, is as unscientific as the refusal to take into account the evidence from good research.

The major response to the often alarming degree of medical practice variations, and the wish to act on evidence from randomised controlled trials, has been the growing enthusiasm for expert protocols and guidelines. Increasingly these are expressed as algorithms, and offered as a more or less safe guide through the maze of confusing variables and their impact on probability.

Although protocols and guidelines are based on evidence from reasearch, the evidence does not always point in the same direction. Nor are the basic building blocks of clinical discourse quite as factual as planners might wish. Estimates in the UK suggest that more than six out of ten presentations of symptoms to GPs cannot be readily "diagnosed"—that is to say interpreted in terms of a recognised pathological process. These clinical problems are not unreal, or unimportant, or insensitive to medical intervention. They are simply diseases without name.

But we are driven to name them. Crombie[2] and his colleagues at the RCGP Research Unit in Birmingham, reviewed the data from the UK second national morbidity study. They found a very wide variation of recording, and showed that for the most part this variation simply reflects the habits of individual doctors—what information they regard as important, what information they chose to exclude from their vision, and what meanings they give. The researchers conclude that, since GPs demonstrated such gross variability in the diagnoses that they chose to name, it will be impossible to use algorithms in the pursuit of desired outcomes.

Risk

Epstein[3] pointed out that the development of guidelines may be especially difficult when patients' preferences are important. Kassirer[4] made similar observations about the need to more explicitly respect patients' preferences in the era of formal guidelines. This became clear to the group considering risk. We reviewed a video programme that permitted patients to consider interventions such as prostatectomy and mastectomy. Whatever the data on effectiveness and efficiency (which can be confusing in relation to both these surgical interventions), individual men were differently threatened by the possibility of postoperative impotence. Women, similarly, were differently affected by the prospect of postoperative mutilation. Given evidence that lumpectomy was as safe as radical mastectomy in her case, one woman opted for the radical procedure on the ground that her breast had betrayed her and she wanted it toally removed. As she spoke, her breast was no longer a part of her body: it had become its enemy.

Criteria of quality

Amongst the group that considered criteria of quality in primary care (chapter 7) there was a great deal of debate about the soundness of the analysis of Londons' problems in the Tomlinson report.[5] At the time of writing, this analysis is coming under mounting attack.[6] The complaint is that the needs of London have been inadequately assessed. But even here, when we come to consider the "fact" of need, we find that data are not morally neutral and can not constitute some sort of impartial judge for the perplexed policy maker. The data speak to our preferences and our beliefs. Willard[7] argued that human needs are not facts (properties, states, processes, relations) about people, but rather are values. He writes: "The attentive observer will probably be amazed at the frequency with which 'need' is employed in discussions and arguments at all levels: common sense, politics, economics, education, morality . . ." Needs, he argues, and specifically medical needs, are in fact wishes or desires on someones part, and are fashioned by the beliefs and values of the wisher. Willard concludes:

> Medical professionals, like the rest of us, must beware of thinking of needs, health or otherwise, as value free facts about people, lest the results of preference, prejudice, professional blindness, failure of moral nerve and social conditioning, parade as the grand and obvious discoveries of objective scientific method.

This seems to me to throw a helpfully clear light on the whole question of need for services. It suggests that the discussion about needs must at the very least embrace an examination of our values and principles, which are an integral part of the evidence from epidemiological studies.

Information

In considering information in an open society (chapter 2) we were much conerned with the quality of information. What was the validity and reliability of the information which we wished to see so widely disseminated? One obvious source of error was the reliability and validity of the raw data collected. Another source of error lay in the interpretation—in the way in which the data were perceived and presented. But there was also an awareness of a more fundamental source, if not of error, then of bias. Attention

7

was thus turned to what sociologists call the "social construction" of information.[8, 9]

Statistics on perinatal mortality, and the report of an inquiry into an avoidable perinatal death in hospital, are different sorts of information but have one key element in common. Both the statistics and the inquiry (the story) are human artefacts, contingencies that cannot be considered as separate from the sources of information—the way in which the information is presented and conveyed. The data are not intellectually or morally neutral. All information suggests answers to questions, either actual or implied by the provider of information. In other words, it is impossible to make a judgment about information, until one asks questions about the reasons for collecting and presenting the information, reasons which may be stated or hidden, intended or unconscious. Thus it is important to be as interested in the questioners as in the answers that they give, because our prejudices and policies may be more powerfully affected by the asking of the question than by the answer to it.

The influence of stakeholders

In almost all six discussion groups that resulted in the following chapters, the question of who were the stakeholders, the major actors in making or influencing policy, was discussed. Richards[10] describes the public service manager as relating to three domains. These she describes as politicians, producers, and consumers. She suggested that the public service manager now needs to relate to all three in what she described as the consumer paradigm of management. The group considering criteria for quality in primary care (chapter 7) were attracted to this model, and adapted it. The three domains were re-labelled government, providers, and consumers. Where Richards linked her three domains by public managers, we linked our three domains of health care by NHS purchasers (fig. 1).

The importance of recognising the particular point of view of each stakeholder became important, when this group began to explore the principles of health care policy, in order to look for criteria by which to evaluate change. A prime example of principles is the list of six dimensions of healthcare quality suggested by Maxwell:[11]

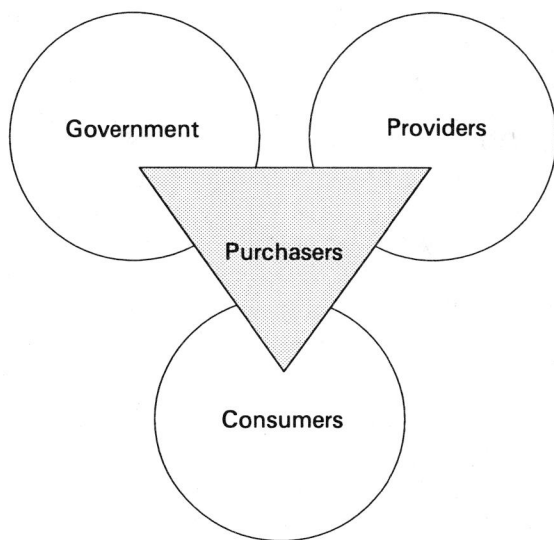

Figure 1   Linking the three domains of health care (after Richards[10]).

- Access to services
- Relevance to need
- Effectiveness
- Equity
- Social acceptability
- Efficiency.

We doubt that all three stakeholders would give the same order of priority to these six principles. To the consumer, the man who fractures his arm at work, the priority may be that he will be seen at once in the A & E department, which would be located near his home. Access and social acceptability would rank highly. For the provider, the surgeon concerned in the case, the effectiveness of his treatment may rank first. For government, concerned to apply limited resources to best effect, efficiency might well take priority over all the rest.

Maxwell himself (personal communication) does not prioritise his dimensions, but offers them as a checklist for judging where a particular provision of service is under-performing. But the point remains that the priority given to principles will depend on the different imperatives of the different players—the different stakeholders.

The impact of complex organisations

In his 1984 article "Who makes the decisions in the NHS?" Klein[12] quoted a model developed by Dunsire[13] to describe complex organisations. This model is characterised by a large multiplicity of vertical axes each representing different policies and professional interests. These vertical axes are intersected by horizontal tiers which represent the different levels of organisation. The model has the appearance of a massive office block. Dunsire writes "The building is a *Tower of Babel* because a different tongue (concepts, vocabulary) is talked on each floor . . . and different jargons and dialects are spoken on any one floor, in each of the corners and other areas."

The impact of language

Dunsire's reference to language throws further light on the differences between stakeholders, and suggests that the facts and the language in which they are expressed, cannot be disentrangled. Once we accept the human identities of our facts, we start to become aware of the languages in which the facts are couched. The facts of the case, the evidence called in support of policies and conclusions, the sense of certainty or uncertainty, are all dependent on the languages that are used. Unless we recognise that each stakeholder expresses principles and policies in a distinctive tongue, we will be confused by the different jargons and dialects which Dunsire observes, and which causes what he calls "linguistic disparity."

The philosopher Richard Rorty[14] said that all languages are contingent (on time, on place, on particular circumstances). We use language in order to create metaphors by which we attempt to understand and manipulate the world in which we find ourselves. In other words the so-called reality of health and health care which each professional recognises is created by the language that he or she has been taught to use. Consequently, Rorty urged irony. By this he meant both a willingness to question the validity and the assumptions built into one's own language, and also a respect for, and an openness to, the languages of others.

Further Rorty suggested that it is impossible successfully to mount a challenge to the validity of ideas expressed in one language, by using the same language. In terms of health care, it is difficult to make a critique the role and function of nursing from within the world of nursing: the same will be true of general practice, of specialist medicine, of public health, and so on. Progress, change, new perceptions will come from the open challenge of one language by another. The key seems to be the development of a mutual respect, and of an expectation of gain from escaping from one's own (limiting) vocabulary of knowledge, skills, and attitudes.

What may be said precisely in one language may become impoverished in another. Greenlanders are said to have an extensive vocabulary to describe a huge variety of conditions of snow. These words refer to texture, consistency, configuration, colour, and much else. However hard the translator tries, no translation can quite capture the nuances of the original. As with all translations, there may be partial failures of accuracy and validity when members of groups or committees seeking to make policy try to communicate.

A GP member of the group considering aging and disease (chapter 5) commented on a passage in the early draft of the chapter which was concerned with biotechnical advance and the possibility of ameliorating or even curing a whole variety of diseases. She observed that in the course of looking at biotechnical possibilities, older people were no longer being described as the subjects of old age, but rather as the objects of medical intervention. The languages of the GP and the professor of geriatrics, both rich in ways of expressing concern for the care of the elderly, by no means shared the same vocabularies or syntax.

Politics and the validity of "facts"

The most often heard criticism of health care policies, including criticisms of the most recent NHS changes, is that they stemmed not from an examination of the facts, but from opinion and political will. The more that we looked for the factual basis of our six topics, the more impressed I became that the facts were neither as solid, nor as reliable, nor as certain as we could have wished. Scepticism in the face of facts is an essential safeguard. Cynicism, that sly and destructive impersonator of scepticism, is dangerous and destructive. Yet it is a paradox that if we do not begin with scepticism, we can be misled into cynicism without ever understanding why.

I would not wish to over-play the relativity of medical facts. The immovable goal remains an evidence based health service, and rationality remains the safest guide to action. Medical research continues to throw new light on diseases and their treatment, which results in impressive progress. Compared with similar social enterprises—the education of our children, the treatment of criminals, the management of the economy—health care can perhaps claim a considerable superiority in the research base of its policy making.

The fact that facts are also values does not invalidate them but infuses them with greater not less meaning. Numerical data have their origin in a human imagination ruled by experience, values, and principles. We cannot safely navigate by the facts as though they were stars, fixed and distant and removed from the interventions of human thought.

Everything that we think and do—the evidence that we rely on for decision making, the courses of action upon which we decide, the criteria against which our actions are to be judged—is deflected through the prism of our values. However meticulous our research and development, however rigorous the collection and interpretation of data, however open and rational our deliberations, unless we pay attention to the moral prism which bends the direction of our thinking, we will constantly miss the point.

The limits of evidence

- Randomised, controlled trials, the gold standard for establishing facts, can determine probability, not outcome

- Patients' choices in relation to risk may be informed by the facts but are also determined by personality and preference

- When facts are determined by stakeholders the research bias may be as much in the questions posed as in the answers obtained

- Facts cannot speak for themselves: like words, they form part of a language which determines a limited range of possible meanings and inferences

---

Paradoxes

Much of the literature on educational assessment deals with the problem of balancing validity and reliability. Essentially validity refers to the closeness of the material under consideration to real life events and experience. In this sense the video recording of GPs' own consultations with patients provide very valid material. Reliability refers to the reproducibility of observations or judgments about these recordings. In terms of an educational assessment, reliability is about fairness to the candidate. The paradox for the examiners who are attempting to assess clinical competence, is that the greater the validity of the test, the more uncertain the reliability. Nothing is more reliable than marking the answers to mutliple choice questionnaires (MCQs), yet MCQs are very far from valid. All examinations are pulled between the polarities of validity and reliability. In all six discussion groups we found ourselves, time and again, pulled between the polarity of alternatives.

In his latest book, *The empty raincoat*, Charles Handy[15] commented on the pervasiveness of paradox in decision making. He described paradoxes as the co-existence of simultaneous opposites, and believes that they do not have to be resolved, only managed. As we found in our discussions, paradoxes are not always opposites, but rather competing goods. Even when they conflict, somehow the very polarity of the paradoxes constitute a sort of unit, a field of discourse. This ambivalence, often at the heart of decision making, is captured in a quotation from the poet Robert Browning, which Handy gives. Browning talks about the paradox that "comforts while it mocks."

The following paradoxes, encountered in the course of our many discussions, illustrate something about the role of paradox in thinking through policies.

Paradoxes

- Elitism and democracy
- Competition and integration
- Beneficience and justice
- Contract and conscience

The paradox of elitism and democracy

In considering criteria for quality in primary care, (chapter 7) we were considering how to evaluate changes consequent on the *Making London better* initiative.[16] We faced the following problem.

In order to achieve the sort of evaluations which we were recommending, the work would have to be carried out with methodological rigour. Since rigorous evluation will be expensive in time, skilled personnel, and other resources, we wanted to recommend that a limited number of key evaluations be identified, and that these should be carried out only by competent academic units.

On the other hand, the very process of evaluation—deliberating about the changes desired, choosing the criteria for judging improvements, determining the best way of looking at these criteria—would have substantial benefit for all those actually involved in developing and delivering the service. In this way, members of a general practice or a community nursing service, would be given a sense of ownership of the changes envisaged, and would themselves create the feedback on their own performance.

Since resources for evaluation must be limited, what would we recommend? Should the resources be widely distributed in order to achieve a sense of general owenrship of the changes? Should we recommend concentration of the resources in academic departments? Would priority be given to the benefits of ownership and participation, or to the benefits of scientific rigour and confidence?

The paradox of competition and integration

Competition between provider units in an internal market is intended to produce greater efficiencies, and a greater sensitivity to the wants of consumers. But the NHS must also be planned, comprehensive, and coherent. No one would suggest that untrammelled competition between rival providers could ever achieve the development of such a planned and integrated national service. This planning and integration is the function of a competent bureaucracy. But bureaucracies, however well staffed, have always been poorly motivated to achieve efficiency, or to be sufficiently sensitive to the wants of consumers. Attempts to reconcile this paradox characterise the current NHS changes.

The group concerned with the availability of information to the public (chapter 2) considered an example which highlights the conflict between the essential characteristics of a market, and the essential values of a public service. A commercial provider of health care, for example a pharmaceutical company, has the right to guard its secrets. The patent laws will protect for many years the intellectual property of a company—the new drugs it has invented. This is essential, since independent companies are in competition with their rivals.

What about the position of the NHS trusts? Trusts too are in competition. Does a trust have the right to keep some of its information secret, in order to maintain a competitive edge? A commercial organisation certainly has such a right. But the trust is both a commercial organisation and an integral part of a public service. Is the public, therefore, not entitled to access to all the (non-personal) information which the trust holds?

The philosopher Jane Jacobs,[17] in her recent book *Systems of survival,* suggests that man has developed two, and only two, systems for surviving in the world. The first, which we share with the animals, she describes as "taking"—making use of what we find around us. Man as a hunter gatherer is the model for this system, which is based on the territorial needs of the tribe. This system of survival gives rise to a morality which she describes as composed of a set of interdependent values. This set of values she calls the "guardian moral syndrome". In the modern world it is translated into the morality of government, the law courts, and the public services.

The second system of survival, unique to human kind, Jacobs describes as trading. Early on man learned to exchange goods, to produce surpluses for exchange, and with this came the growth of manufacture, business, and the mercantile society. This trading system came to be equally well served by its own set of interdependent moral precepts. These precepts she describes as the "commercial moral syndrome".

The moral precepts in each of the two syndromes seem to be paired. And the pairs always contradict one another. In the guardian syndrome, largesse and adherence to tradition are virtues; in the commercial, thrift and openness to novelty. Each group of precepts, however, is internally consistent and results in social benefit.

If I read Jacobs aright, then the activities of the NHS fall into both categories or syndromes. The work of the Department of Health and the purchasing authorities, the pursuit of Health of the Nation, are driven by the values of the guardian moral syndrome. The work of health care providers (general practices, hospital trusts, medical research units, pharmaceutical companies) are driven by the values of the commercial moral syndrome.

Jacobs suggests that the danger lies in carelessly mixing the two sets of values. The examples she gives from North America are the intrusion of government into business enterprises, and the attempt to organise public services as though they were private companies. She argues that it is possible to create a successful synergy between the two sets of values—but this has to be done with great sensitivity to the essential differences between them. In the NHS we are being challenged to find a new synergy between the private and public ownership of information.

The paradox of beneficience and justice

Among other things, in considering risk, we were considering the impact of lifestyles on health chances. A surgeon in the North of England had been reported as refusing to perform a coronary artery bypass graft on a middle-aged man who was a heavy smoker. Was this a reasonable way of handling risk in medicine? Two questions arose. Firstly, what is the citizen's entitlement from public funds for the treatment of a condition deemed to be a consequence of the patient's own risk taking behaviour? Secondly, what would constitute a reasonable response by this surgeon?

For a number of reasons we could say that the *ab initio* refusal of treatment is not morally sustainable. Coronary artery disease is the result not simply of risky behaviour, but of the interaction between the behaviour and the patient's particular genetic make-up. Most diseases have very complex and interacting causes, many of them outside the control of the individual patient. Moreover the ability to give up smoking, to control diet, and so on depends on the availability of these choices. The decision to stop smoking and reduce weight is arguably much more available to relatively affluent middle class persons, than to an unemployed and relatively impoverished individual who has had a poor education and domestic environment.

On the other hand, the surgeon who demands that his patient cooperate in his treatment is surely behaving reasonably. In this case the unwillingness of the patient to cooperate (to give up smoking) was now a deliberate rejection of an available choice, and materially increased the likelihood of an unfavourable outcome to the coronary bypass surgery. By incurring an additional but avoidable risk the patient was greatly reducing the likely benefit of surgery. The surgeon was therefore simply trying to balance individual justice with distributive justice. He decided to use the limited resources available to him in order to purchase material benefit for others, at the expense of the very marginal benefit of this particular and uncooperative individual.

Two sorts of justice, parallel and conflicting, produce another paradox that has to be managed.

The paradox of contract and conscience

Throughout the developed world two irreconcilable forces are shaping health services:

- The intention to bring all citizens within the safety net of assured health care either from public funds or private insurance
- The escalating cost of this care as biotechnology advances and public expectation increases.

The policy response to this paradox, both in the NHS and abroad, has been the advent of managed health care.

However idealistic the commitment of government or health maintenance organisations or other insurance based provider, to access, effectiveness, equity, and so on, efficiency is perhaps the most obvious intention of public policy. For, whatever level of funding is deemed nationally affordable or politically expedient, there is a responsibility to achieve the best possible value for money.

The major consequence of this has been the increasing replacement of professional medical opinion and power, in the shaping of the health service, by management—by the drawing up of contractual obligations. Although contracts may be much concerned with the whole range of Maxwell's six dimensions, they are ultimately driven by the imperative of efficiency.

Doctors, nurses and other healthcare professionals now have to function in what has been described as a new "age of contract".[18] Examples abound: the purchasing contracts between health authorities and trusts; the clinical protocols and guidelines discussed earlier in this chapter; the specific targets for

17

preventive medicine measures which are now built into the GPs' remuneration package; the monetary control of prescribing—limited lists and indicative budgets. Even the continuing education of GPs, an activity which might be considered to be of the essence of professionalism, is now controlled by the quite detailed determinants of the postgraduate educational allowance.

In considering rational prescribing (chapter 6), we were of course much concerned with the whole range of quality considerations. But no group of professionals, whether they are concerned with making policy or, as here, with reflecting about policy, exists in a social vacuum. Much of the discussion, therefore, was dominated by issues of efficiency—although efficient prescribing is reflected not only in cost benefit but also in the avoidance of unnecessary prescribing and iatrogenic damage.

The reform of prescribing habits is deemed necessary by almost all of the stakeholders concerned—government, the pharmaceutical industry, and the medical profession—although each of these stakeholders have a different view about how the habits should change. The attempts to reform prescribing in the NHS now throws the sharpest light on the paradox of contract and conscience.

Changes in prescribing may be brought about by restriction—for example, by creating a limited list of drugs in a particular therapeutic category; by the encouragement of generic (non-patent and usually cheaper) equivalents; by creating indicative prescribing budgets. These regulations can be, and often are, reinforced by training. Training may be described as the preparation of the learner to respond in a particular and approved manner to a precisely predicted situation. The doctor can be trained to respond to condition A with drug X in one situation, and drug Y in another. These managerial and training measures work—that is to say, they have been demonstrated to achieve their objectives of reducing expenditure. What they cannot in themselves achieve is discriminating and effective prescribing.

Education, in contrast with training, is the preparation of the learner to respond in a logical but creative way, to unpredicted situations. Education, therefore, can prepare the doctor to emabrace real therapeutic innovations and advances so as to bring the best care to patients, while retaining a robust scepticism for the claims of pharmaceutical companies. The prerequisites of such an attitude to the changing therapeutic oportunities, is that the doctors understand the underlying biological arguments, and are able to judge the scientific quality of trials. Overwhelmingly doctors are trained, not educated, to treat their patients. Training serves the imperative of contract—compliant behaviour. Education serves the imperative of professionalism—the exercise of judgment.

Without training and contract the NHS would become financially and managerially unsustainable. Without education and professional judgment the doctor's response to the patient would become increasingly unreflective, rigid, and inappropriate. Somehow the paradox has to be managed.

Consensus

During an early think tank meeting, one of the members, true to his academic provenance, suggested that we should begin with a comprehensive literature search and review. Another member, no less academically oriented, suggested that this would be inappropriate: we were not engaged in "that kind of activity". What kind of activity were we engaged in? What light would our deliberation throw on the way in which policies emerge?

The six groups had no formal mandates, authorities or lines of accountability which would have permitted the making of policy. We were not committees. Although we functioned under the aegis of respected national organisations, they were our sponsors, and we were not their servants or even their consultants. Our task was to explore some of the scientific, moral and societal dimensions of certain aspects of health care policy which were of mutual interest. In each group an expert writer was identified and charged with the task of producing the relevant chapter in this book. To what extent would these chapters (which were to go through several drafts, which would be commented on by all the group members) represent a consensus?

At the outset it was clear that, however influenced by different members of the group, the writer accepts responsibility for what is written. Consequently, what is written in the following chapters may include ideas or materials which different members might have expressed differently, or from which they would have wished to distance themselves. To complicate matters further, each think tank functioned in its own idiosyncratic way. One writer might firmly take the chair, and exercise the weight of professional authority or scientific or managerial expertise. Another would act as a facilitator, looking for areas of agreement, seeking to move the group in concert towards the completion of the task. Is this how policies emerge from government, from purchasing authorities, and from boards of trusts? Are policies the result of consensus among those charged with the responsibility for making them? What is consensus, how is it achieved, and who are its constituents members?

The raw material of policy making is derived from evidence and values. Earlier in this chapter I suggested the substantial overlap between the two. A consideration of evidence and values reveals a simultaneous and parallel existence of different and more or less competing goods—the paradoxes that need to be managed. The management of these paradoxes brings into play a variety of human forces. These include the individual characteristics of the policy makers—their personalities, their styles of behaviour, their sense of role, their beliefs about science and society, and so on. But since all policy results from interactions between people, policy must also be substantially shaped by the nature of group interaction.

The Delphi technique,[19] much used in determining clinical policies, attempts to remove as far as possible the effects of group dynamics on decision taking. The opinions of large groups of experts are elicited by postal questionnare. Questionnaires are re-circulated a number of times, the answers increasingly falling where the weight of opinion is accumulating, until in subsequent questionnaires there is a convergence on what can be taken as a consensus view. In place of group dynamics, consensus appears to be achieved by impersonal and therefore relatively unbiased methods. But such consensus here has much more to do with the social imperative of solidarity, than with the truth.

Our six think tanks relied on group discussion. Although they differed much in the objects of discourse and the personalities of their members, they were engaged not in committee work but in small group work. Reflecting on this, and my experience elsewhere in committees, I developed the following tentative model, contrasting characteristics, tasks, consequences, dominant values, and end points (Table I). This exaggerates the differences between groups and committees, but suggests something about the uncertain nature of consensus in policy making.

Members of small groups are not selected by democratic or

TABLE I Differences between small group work and committee work.

	Group work	Committee work
Characteristics	Social Internal affiliation Task oriented	Political External affiliations Result oriented
Tasks	Explore differences Define paradox	Decide goals Reach agreement
Consequences	Focus on principles Set limits to compromise	Focus on actions Generate rules
Dominant values	Beneficence Autonomy Advocacy	Non-maleficence Efficiency Justice
End points	Judgment	Compliance

bureaucratic processes. They tend to be self selected, or brought together by an individual or sponsoring institution. They interact socially, that is to say their personal values and prejudices are close to the surface of their deliberations. The commitment is to the group and its processes, and to this extent the affiliation may be described as internal.

Committee members are either elected or chosen to be representatives or delegates so that their own personal views must be adapted to the policies or interests of those whom they represent. Therefore their personal values and prejudices, although almost always in evidence, must be constantly subordinated to the committee's tasks. Interpersonal differences become political differences. The affiliations of the committee members are external.

Members engaged in group work are free to explore and define the paradoxes which abound, to examine them in terms of the principles which the members bring to the work. Consequently, the values that dominate group work tend to be the more obviously liberal and permissive ones of beneficence, autonomy, and advocacy. The intention of group work is to produce judgment.

Committee members, when they encounter paradoxes, are enjoined to decide between them, sometimes even to vote. The job of the committee is to reach agreement, to take action, and to generate rules. The values which dominate committee work therefore tend to be the more conservative and restrictive ones of non-maleficence, efficiency, and justice. The intention of committee work is to produce compliance.

The members of our think tanks did not have to reach agreement about anything. Their task was exploration—an opening up of possibilities, not the foreclosures of options. This kind of work is not part of policy making, but it may be a necessary precondition for soundness.

The recent turbulence surrounding the NHS changes in the 1990s has yet again raised the question of whether there is still a moral consensus about the future of the service. If we are to talk about such a moral consensus, we will have to examine the prerequisite of such consensus—compromise. At one extreme consensus can be described as the core of values that remain after all the nuances and contradictions that stem from our different cultures, our experiences, our roles, and our personalities have been stripped away. Such a consensus is a *reductio ad absurdum*; a collection of anodyne decisions which do not matter to any of the decision makers. At the other extreme, consensus is a measure of the degree to which all the parties concerned are prepared to sacrifice what they really believe and want, in the name of professional, or other social solidarity. Such mutually resented compromise can only produce paper agreements without effective action.

Compromise can be expressed both negatively and positively. In its negative sense, compromise suggests an absence of principles, a commitment to short term gain, to self interest, to retaining power without purpose. In its positive sense, compromise speaks of reasonableness, sensitivity to the limits of ones own understanding, to what Rorty describes as the contingency of the languages that each of us uses. Without such positive compromise there can be no real solidarity, no truly democratic government, and no effective, efficient, and just policy making.

Conclusions

These reflections on the chapters to follow, on the processes that went into their making, are of course entirely personal and idiosyncratic. There is no attempt at consensus here, however defined and understood. The lesson that I take from my membership of the six groups is that at all levels of policy making, we need to pay increasing attention to the nature of evidence, the pervasiveness of paradox and the many modes of consensus.

The fact that facts are also values, that principles are also paradoxes, does not diminish but rather enhances them. It also transforms them, reveals them to be a part of the dialectic. Facts and principles are often presented as the yardsticks by which the rightness or morality of the dialogue may be judged. But in debate, when facts and principles are used only as yardsticks, they are transformed into weapons in a struggle that turns on strength and skill, not on reason and justice.

Much of the literature on consensus in medicine refers to the function of ethics committees.[20] This is helpful, since what Handy calls the management of paradox is little different from what medical ethicists have called the resolution of dilemmas. Jennings[21] urges us to think of consensus not as a thing, or a goal, but rather an activity. He regrets the lack of a gerund form of the word, in English—"consensing". He says: "Consensus should enjoy moral weight in decision making only when we are satsified that consensus reflects a health community of open, inclusive moral discovery and growth."

So much of the debate on health care policy seems to rest on the special pleading of interested parties where evidence is selectively used as a weapon, paradox paraded as ideological struggle, and consensus as the moral imperative of whichever party (political or professional) is presenting its case.

In examining information in an open society, chapter 2 makes a strong argument for openness of information. With this must go a broadly based discussion about the provenance of this information, what warning it contains, and what promises it holds out. The broadcast media have special responsibility here. For such a democratic moral discourse to take place, we will require forums for debate and exploration rather different from those which we have inherited. I hope that this book will make some modest contribution to the growth of such discourse.

References

1 Hills G. The knowledge disease. *BMJ* 1993; 307: 1578.
2 Crombie DL, Cross KW, Fleming DM. The problem of diagnostic variability in general practice. *J Epidemiol Community Health* 1992; 46: 447–54.

3 Epstein AM 1990. The outcome movement—will it get us where we want to go? *N Engl J Med* 1992; **323**(4): 266–9.

4 Kassirer JP. Incorporating patients preferences into medical decisions. *N Engl J Med* 1994; **330**; 1895–6.

5 The Tomlinson Report. *Report of the enquiry into London's health service, medical education and research.* London: HMSO, 1992.

6 Jarman B. Is London over-bedded? *BMJ* 1993; **306**: 979–82.

7 Willard LD. Needs and medicine. *J Med Phil* 1982; 7(3): 259–73.

8 Shaw M, Miles I. 1979. The social roots of statistical knowledge. In: Irvine J, Miles I, Evans J, editors. *Demystifying social statistics.* London: Pluto Press.

9 Armstrong D. The invention of infant mortality. *Sociol Health Illness* 1986; **8**(3): 211–32.

10 Richards S. *Public Managers in the middle: working paper.* Public Management Foundation, 1994.

11 Maxwell RJ. Quality assessment in health. *BMJ* 1984; **288**: 1470–2.

12 Klein R. Who makes the decisions in the NHS? *BMJ* 1984; **288**: 1706–8.

13 Dunsire A. Implementation in a bureaucracy. Oxford: Martin Robertson, 1978.

14 Rorty R. *Contingency, irony and solidarity.* Cambridge: Cambridge University Press, 1989.

15 Handy C. *The empty raincoat.* London: Hutchinson, 1994.

16 Department of Health. *Making London better.* London: Department of Health, 1993.

17 Jacobs J. *Systems of survival.* London: Hodder & Stoughton, 1992.

18 Bevan G, Marinker M. *Greening the White Paper.* London: Social Market Foundation, 1990.

19 Russell I, Grimshaw J, Wilson B. *Proc R Soc Edinburgh,* 1993; **101B**.

20 Veatch RM, Moreno JD. Consensus in panels and committees: conceptual and ethical issues. *J Med Phil* 1991; **16**(4); 371–4.

21 Jennings B. Possibilities of consensus: toward democratic discourse. *J Med Phil* 1991; **16**(4): 462.

Chapter 2
What sort of information should be available to the public in an open society?

Julia Neuberger

Partner: THE SOCIAL MARKET FOUNDATION

By and large the so called facts about medicine and health care are presented in a rather sensational way—by doctors, policy analysts, managers, party politicians, and journalists. Should there be a public policy of providing information which is as accurate and informative as possible? Should this involve information not only about what medical care can achieve, but also what it can not achieve?

Author:	Rabbi Julia Neuberger	*Chairman, Camden and Islington Community Health Services NHS Trust*
Convener:	Professor Marshall Marinker	
Members:	Mr Mark Bassett	*Health Policy Adviser, SMF*
	Dr Ken Burch	*General Practitioner, Oxford*
	Professor Cyril Chantler	*Principal, United Medical and Dental Schools of Guy's and St Thomas's*
	Dr David Colin-Thomé	*General Practitioner/ Fundholder, Cheshire*
	Mr Danny Finkelstein	*Director, The Social Market Foundation*
	Lord Kilmarnock	*Editorial Director, The Social Market Foundation*
	Dr Rod Sheaff	*Fellow in Health Service Management, University of Manchester*

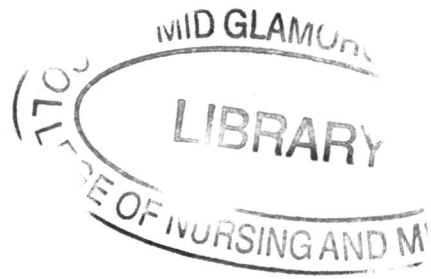

Introduction

A healthcare system which is publicly funded has a duty to be open about its decision making, its resource allocation policy, and its priorities. This is a requirement of good governance, but it also properly tips the balance away from those who provide or purchase health care to the users of those services. For information is power. The informed citizen can ask a variety of questions of government and of public, voluntary, and private providers of goods and services if, and only if, she or he has a sufficient base on which to build and phrase questions in such a way as to get data that will be useful in making a specific decision.

In the field of health care, that could be personal—about whether to proceed with a particular intervention, or to allow a child or very elderly relative to do so. Or, rather differently, it could be of wider public interest, where decisions are made by purchasers of health care, perhaps with government guidance, about what health care to buy on behalf of a community.

The degree to which an individual can participate in this decision making, both personal and community based, is governed precisely by the amount of information to which he or she has access, and the extent to which that has been made available in a form sufficiently intelligible to be helpful within the debate. This kind of open debate is somewhat foreign to the NHS, which has hitherto been centrally driven and is now moving towards being decentralised and increasingly purchaser driven. But whether such openness should be welcomed depends on the political views of any given group. There is an argument for information to be made freely available in order for the market to work efficiently; for with restricted access to information the purchasers, providers, and users of services cannot make the proper choices essential to a market system. But there is also a view which regards free flow of information as dangerous, making it more difficult to provide health care for people in an organised way.

Countering objections to making information available

The principle stands, of making all information available unless a very good reason can be adduced for not doing so.

Administrative difficulty is not a sufficient objection. Nor, indeed, is cost, since it could be argued that the cost of making information available is a necessary cost in a market system. Within the NHS, this is complicated by the fact that the purchasers are not the actual users of services, making it an inexact market. The costs of providing the information and the benefits gained from its provision are not necessarily borne by the same people, and there are some who would argue that making all the information available could lead to overconsumption of a free good. However, there is no possibility of making informed choices for purchasers or users without the information, so the principle must stand that all information be made available, recognising that the effects of such openness would be considerable. If information is power, then such a policy of transparency would transfer power away from healthcare professionals to patients, and demystify healthcare interventions. It would also transfer power from government and civil servants to citizens, and it would answer, at least to some extent, through the open decision making that would then have to ensue, the criticism of the new membership of NHS health authorities and trust boards, that they are unelected. For, if these appointed bodies were required to be wholly accountable for their decisions, and to be transparent about how they reached them, considerable power would rest with ordinary citizens and, in the case of the NHS, increasingly with community health councils and other patient groups.

Nevertheless, a wider public debate needs to be held about the internal market. For there is real conflict in the new reformed NHS between the argument that calls for openness in public services, and requires open government for good governance, and the argument that providers have to be able to keep some of their innovations, prices, and advantages secret in order to be better able to compete with neighbouring providers, both in the public and private sector. In other words, if the competition to provide rests between public, voluntary, and private sector bodies, then the fact that some are in the public sector should not place upon them a greater duty of openness than that which applies to the private sector, which can claim a need for commercial confidentiality as a reason for not revealing everything to all its competitors. Since the principle of openness must prevail over this argument, however, the requirement must be for any body providing services funded by public monies, be they in the private, voluntary, or public sector, to be open about its decision making. Such organisations could even be required to disseminate information about their services, outcomes, and quality indicators, for instance, on request.

We have assumed that we are talking about health services purchased with public money largely, but not wholly, in the public domain. And it is for this reason that we argue that the citizen is entitled to any information that can be reasonably made available to him or her, in the field of health care, unless there are compelling reasons, such as patient confidentiality or early planning disclosure, why that should not be so. There are many examples of information being kept confidential in the sectional interest of a particular professional or management group, such as data on perioperative deaths, which surgeons would prefer not to be released into the public domain. Other examples might be competitive pricing data between provider units, as mentioned earlier, or mortality statistics between one provider unit and another, which the public might well want to know.

Problems of data interpretation

Comparative mortality statistics are a good example of a situation in which medical and managerial staff are resistant to the information being made available, using the argument that, with such wide variance in case-mix, the data are too complicated for general public consumption. Such an argument has to be taken seriously, yet should not stop the provision of information of this kind. The very real fears on the part of various professionals, that they are going to be judged on the basis of their performance in what might be a rather a crude way, need to be recognised. So a warning of considerable generality in the data might need to be given to its users.

Statistics on perinatal mortality, and the report of an enquiry into an avoidable perinatal death in hospital, are further examples of sorts of information not necessarily easy for the public at large to interpret. They have one key element in common. Both the statistics and the enquiry are human artefacts, and cannot be considered separately from the sources of information, the way in which the information is presented and conveyed, and the fact that, though raw facts are neutral, data as collected are not intellectually or morally neutral, since their very method of collection is likely to be influenced by a desire to answer some

29

particular question. It is impossible to make a judgment about information until one asks questions about the reasons for collecting and presenting it, reasons which may be either stated or hidden, intended or unconscious.

It is therefore legitimate to ask:

- What was the purpose of gathering the information, such as examining cross-infection rates in the hope that something might be done about them
- Who asked for it, such as the government looking at prescribing habits of GPs in order to examine whether it would be possible to cut the drugs bill
- Who collected, collated, and reported it
- What stakes these people or organisations have in the questions and answers
- What sort of information is being dealt with: stories, observations, enquiries, data sets, and so on
- How the information was produced, including the research methods, the rigour involved, and the standard of monitoring
- To what extent the information as produced is already the subject of interpretation
- Whether the information is presented in the shape of conclusions rather than raw data from which an individual can draw his or her own conclusions
- What information is missing in a story, and whether omissions were accidental or intended.

It is therefore critical that we begin to define what information is, or at least provide an adequate framework for categorising it, so that it is easy to ask questions about who provided the information, or decided to withhold it, for what purpose and for whom, and how it was produced. There are various categories of information which intersect, but they fall into two broad categories:

- That which allows individuals and organisations (such as patients and purchasers) to make personal or corporate choices (on behalf of a company, for instance)
- That which allows us to participate fully as citizens within a democratic community in the public debate about health care policy and expenditure.

Organisational and resourcing aspects

It is not possible to have a rational debate about proper use of NHS monies and prioritisation without far greater information about what is available, what is effective, and where regional and local variations lie. Instead of clinical freedoms, so called, which are in fact clinical prejudices, there should be comprehensive information about effectiveness available, such as that produced by the Nuffield Institute at Leeds (UK Clearing House on Health Outcomes, Nuffield Institute, University of Leeds)

At present, it is virtually impossible to get much of this information. Parliament has become an inadequate forum for information about the NHS. Questions asked by backbench members of parliament produce all too frequently the reply that this information is not held centrally. It could be argued that this is a form of censorship imposed by government, for there is as yet no duty upon NHS trusts to collect some of these data locally, or for local purchasing organisations to have to answer questions locally. Such a duty, clearly recognised, would help local residents and could be immediately responsive to local concerns, bypassing the cumbersome and often ineffective parliamentary procedure. If there are worries about information being held so locally as to make a national debate about resource allocation virtually impossible, these must be addressed, perhaps by requiring all local answers to be lodged with the information watchdog, as recommended later.

The spectre of disproportionate use of resources in information retrieval for certain bodies cannot help but be present. Yet it must be the case that it is a legitimate use of resources, though in the view of some people not necessarily optimum, to help to create better information systems and good access to them. It is therefore legitimate to take money away from direct health care if it is necessary in order to increase information availability, particularly if it can be demonstrated that better access to information encourages better use of the services available—including sometimes the decision not to use services at all. The overall cost of such information provision would be small in comparison with general expenditure, and the added possibility of greater local efficiency being of real benefit in cost and accountability terms makes it an attractive option. Indeed, proper information might well lead people to use the services of the NHS more discriminatingly and more efficiently.

Open information: types and uses

Types of information that should be available

It might be possible to construct rules which would distinguish between information in a variety of ways so that, for instance, different questions would be asked of and safeguards applied to information attributable to organisations, institutions, or individuals from those applied to information which is non-attributable or where ownership of the information is unclear. An informed debate about what information is available, or should be, might then ensue.

The health information in which we are interested should include:

- Epidemiological profiles, including variance in incidence nationally and internationally, as well as local data on deprivation and details of calculations for weighted capitation for health spending
- Comparative outcomes data, so patients and purchasers can choose amongst the available options where they go for treatment, and what they receive. Examples might include Walter Holland's *Atlas of avoidable mortality*[1] for general information, with added data about variance in outcomes from breast cancer, as demonstrated by the South East Thames Cancer Registry, or the fourfold variation of survival in colonic cancer from Glasgow Health Board. The Royal College of Surgeons' data on perioperative deaths might also be included here
- Risk versus benefit in certain procedures or interventions, including far better drug information for patients, as advocated by RADAR-UK
- Clinical profiles of care
- Information about human biology
- Information about current research, especially about that research (some 5%) which is abandoned and never sees the light of day because it does not show what its funders wanted to prove. One key improvement would be a requirement upon researchers who invite patients to participate in trials as research subjects to inform those patients, or indeed healthy volunteers, of the results of the trial in which they participated
- Information about public expenditure policy, health economics, and cost-benefit ratios

> ## Types of information that should be available
>
> - Epidemiological profiles and details of calculations for weighted capitation for health spending
> - Comparative outcomes data
> - Risk-benefit information on procedures and drugs
> - Clinical profiles of care
> - Information on human biology
> - Research results, including projects that are abandoned
> - Public expenditure policy, health economics, and cost-benefit ratios
> - Social, economic, and environmental determinants of health

- Information on non-NHS determinants of health, including such examples as water and air quality, smoking research, environmental pollution, occupational health hazards, poverty, income distribution, and housing.

All that having been said, although the precise definition of information may often elude us, the overriding principle for all involved in the field of health care is that there is "transparency" about information in the public domain. This is essential for the proper functioning of a democratic system. The onus, therefore, is upon the person or organisation who wishes to withhold information to prove a necessity to do so. That may now include the private sector, since members of private healthcare schemes are now some 12% of the population.

Uses for information

On all these counts the argument goes strongly in favour of the giving of information in order that:

- The citizen may be more able to influence policy formation
- The consumer/patient/user can know (a) the range of services and how to gain access to them, and (b) something on outcomes, risks, and conditions caused by medical intervention
- Good practice can be widely disseminated, and innovations discussed and publicised

- Transparent monitoring of policy can take place, especially controversial or official policy that government or other agencies are unwilling to implement effectively, such as where particular rhetoric has been used about patient choice but that choice has actually diminished. An example would be the difficulty of getting an extracontractual referral for a patient outside the purchaser's or GP fundholder's normal contract, even though this is what the patient might well prefer.
- Expression can be given to cases where consumers/patients/users are deceived, where corruption takes place, or where material evidence on health care, consumer goods, and drugs is misrepresented or concealed.

Underlying these demands for information is the view that an open information policy is a corrective to:

- Government and civil service interests in concealing or obfuscating data (for example, waiting list data, where people have been taken off a waiting list that is too long)
- Commercial bodies' interest in concealing data on quality, safety, or alternatives to their products, plus corresponding data on competing products. This applies both to the private sector and to the public sector, whether commercial or quasicommercial bodies (for example NHS trusts) are involved
- Professionals' resistance to revealing their professional mysteries and demystifying their practice
- Managers—especially the "traditional public sector stereotype"—avoiding intellectually challenging or politically controversial issues
- The information imbalance that always exists between healthcare personnel, especially doctors, and their patients.

All the above rests upon an assumption that the exchange or giving of information places responsibilities upon both the giver and the recipient. This applies in all relationships—between patient and professional, provider and purchaser, NHS and government. Each side has a responsibility to ask sensible questions and to ask for information that is readily available. Each side also has a responsibility to deal sensitively with the answers, which implies a level of equality of relationship as yet unknown in the NHS.

Catechisms: a mode for conveying information

However, information is only useful, beyond acting as a corrective to power bases, if it provides helpful answers to pertinent questions and has the capacity to lead to clear benefit for users. How to frame questions about a variety of issues within the health service becomes an issue of paramount importance. Indeed, we would recommend a series of "catechisms", which people could use in a wide variety of circumstances, such as by a patient who has been referred to hospital, or for whom a particular drug has been prescribed, or who has been invited to participate in a clinical trial. A patient example might run something like the one given below.

Obviously, both patients and doctors would have to learn to use this form of catechism, but it is clear that it could be very valuable, like the Consumers for Ethics in Research (CERES) series of questions for patients being asked to enter a clinical trial[2] or David Sackett's simple series of questions for clinicians to distinguish between useful and useless or harmful therapy.[3] This system is not hard to develop, although such lists of questions would have to be tested out.

Similarly, purchasers could develop a series of catechisms to ask of their providers, such as how calculations of costs are made, how quality of services is assured, the extent to which users of services are consulted about the times and days

---

Example of a "catechism" for patients

- What would be the likely outcome without treatment?
- What is the objective/effectiveness of each treatment?
- What are the alternative treatments?
- What treatment targets will be set?
- What are the most common side effects or interactions?
- When should one stop, change intensity, or switch treatment?
- Is it cheaper to prescribe privately or to buy over the counter?
- Would the doctor use the same treatment on him/herself or family?
- Where did the doctor get his/her information about the drug?

of services, the use of temporary and agency staff, and so on, some of which is already done by the Audit Commission. Providers, meanwhile, ought to be able to ask purchasers a series of questions about the extent to which they are genuinely interested in quality, or whether cost is of paramount importance, about how the purchasers will monitor quality, about the extent to which the users' concerns are genuinely taken into account, and what user surveys have shown.

An information culture

It is demonstrably possible, as pilot projects have shown, and clearly desirable, to inculcate a culture of information provision and questioning into all health service relationships. This in itself would open up the service to the public gaze, but it would also transform individual relationships, removing at least part of the old paternalistic relationship between professionals who "know best" and patients who are expected simply to accept what they are given. It would enable a decision making process to come into being which is considerably more informed, at all levels, and above all "transparent".

That transparency could in fact be tested by some form of audit. There could be an agency or agencies charged with the collection, collation, and maintenance of data sets, as well as the commissioning of studies in order to obtain information, interpret it, and disseminate it. But this would be yet another form of quango. It might be more sensible, and simpler, to give a much more limited sampling and watchdog role to the Audit Commission, which has already commented in detail on the lamentable lack of information and poor quality of communications within the NHS.[4, 5]

The cost of such information provision will not be negligible. But, without it, the public will feel increasingly dissatisfied with the governance of the NHS, and feel increasingly excluded from the decision making process, on both a personal and a corporate level. Therefore it is right to argue that some expenditure on making information available to those who require it, within certain constraints, is a necessary part of sensible healthcare funding.

Dilemmas: confidentiality and regulation

Confidentiality

There are dilemmas in all this. One key issue lies in the field of innovation, for instance, when there are competing bodies, not necessarily wholly or all commercial. In order to reward innovation one must be able to attribute new intellectual property to its inventor, and direct rewards to the inventor alone. But the public interest lies in rapid dissemination of, say, life saving innovations. Commercial sensitivity alone cannot therefore be a defence against providing information in a publicly funded healthcare system.

Equally, in all this argument for transparency, personal information about patients should always be excluded from an open information policy on the grounds that there has to be very good reason why any personal and identifying information about individuals should ever reach the public domain at all (see box), though individuals should be able to access their own health records to a greater extent that the Access to Health Records Act 1991 requires.

But in all this there are uncertain areas, such as which intra-organisation information (that is, managerial information) should rightly be in the public domain—market testing results? information to support bargaining? costing? discussion documents?

Exclusions from an open information policy

- Health records, including PAS-type data on the fact of receiving psychiatric treatment or being "sectioned" under the Mental Health Act, contraceptive services, treatment of sexually transmitted diseases (even where there may be a risk to partners of the patient), and occupational disease

- Matters being investigated by the police or *sub judice*

- Information on adoption, fostering, family therapy, infertility services, care proceedings for children, and any related social work

- Information covered by a doctor's duty of confidentiality

- Personal employment and health information

- Prison or criminal records, subject to the principles enshrined in the Rehabilitation of Offenders Act

---

Regulation

If the Audit Commission is charged with sampling the availability of information in the NHS, there is still a problem of regulation and implementation in all this. Should there be, for example, a public right of access to unpublished data from non-governmental organisations, such as private healthcare providers? It might be an acid test of the bona fides of private healthcare organisations if they were prepared to submit themselves to such a requirement. Should it be possible to ensure that the public is informed of useful services which have been withdrawn, or of services which are of unproven outcome yet continue to be offered to the public, or about services which may be useful but are not yet being made available?

Some method of registering what data are held where and how to access them is essential, as is public access to knowledge of where data are held in their least interpreted (most original or "raw") forms. It ought to be possible to map out where gaps lie in the present plethora of information to be found in the public domain and whether its absence is accidental or deliberate. Then, to continue the transparency argument, it should be possible to argue for all that information to be made available, unless a good reason for not doing so is put forward. Pressing this point, with a particular agency (for example, the Audit Commission) charged with doing so, should enable the NHS to change its culture and make information available, and discourage it from doing useless or even dangerous things. Indeed, should the Audit Commission find something terribly wrong with the information available, or not being made available, anywhere within publicly funded health care, it should make this the subject of a separate report.

Summary and recommendations

Information is an integral part both of a managed organisation, and a free market. The NHS is a national organisation which should therefore provide its information, whether locally or nationally, in the same way everywhere. There should be a common accounting system, clearly understood by all concerned, and common quality standards, for without these the public cannot hope to begin to understand what is being compared with what. The NHS Management Executive should be charged with ensuring that this happens, and that purchasers and providers have a duty to make information available to the public on a transparent, right-to-know, basis.

The minimum required changes to put some of this into effect, a summary of our recommendations, include:

- It should be a requirement for any body providing services funded by public monies, be they in the private, voluntary, or public sector, to be open about their decision making. They should be required to disseminate information about their services, outcomes, and quality indicators, for instance, on request
- There should be an entitlement for the citizen to any information that can be reasonably made available to him or her, in the field of health care, unless there are compelling reasons, such as patient confidentiality or early planning disclosure, why that should not be so
- There should be a duty upon NHS trusts to collect some of these data locally, and for local purchasing organisations to have to answer questions locally
- Lest such local accountability makes a national debate about resource allocation virtually impossible, all local answers should be lodged with the information watchdog.
- The overriding principle for all involved in the field of health care is that there is "transparency" about information in the public domain. The onus, therefore, is upon the person or organisation who wishes to withhold information to prove a necessity to do so. The argument goes strongly in favour of the giving of information in order that:
  —the citizen can influence policy formation
  —the consumer/patient/user will be better informed about services
  —good practice and innovations can be widely disseminated
  —transparent monitoring of policy can take place
  —expression can be given to cases of deception of consumers, corruption, and misrepresentation or concealment of evidence on health care
- We would recommend a series of catechisms which people could use in a wide variety of circumstances, such as by a

patient who is referred to hospital, or for whom a particular drug has been prescribed, or who has been invited to participate in a clinical trial

- A limited sampling and watchdog role over information should be given to the Audit Commission, which has already commented in detail on the lamentable lack of information, and poor quality communications, within the NHS
- Some expenditure on making information available to those who require it, within certain constraints, is a necessary part of sensible healthcare funding
- Some method of registering what data are held where and how to access them is essential, as is public access to knowledge of where data are held in their least interpreted (most original or "raw") forms. It ought to be possible, by this approach, to map out where gaps lie in the present plethora of information to be found in the public domain and whether its absence is accidental or deliberate
- Should the Audit Commission find something terribly wrong with the information available, or not being made available, anywhere within publicly funded health care, it should make this the subject of a separate report
- There should be a common accounting system, clearly understood by all concerned, and common quality standards,

---

A summary of the recommendations

- Dissemination of information by all service providers
- Patients' entitlement to information
- A duty for NHS trusts to collect and supply information locally
- An information watchdog role for the Audit Commission
- A culture of "transparency" for information in the public domain
- Development of "catechisms" for obtaining information
- Recognition that expenditure on making information available is a necessity
- A central register of what data are held where, and how they can be accessed
- Common information standards instituted by the NHS Executive

---

for without these the public cannot hope to begin to understand what is being compared with what. The NHS Management Executive should be charged with ensuring that this happens and that purchasers and providers have a duty to make information available to the public on a transparent, right-to-know, basis

References

1 Holland W W. *European Community atlas of avoidable death*. Vols 1 and 2. Oxford: Oxford University Press, (Health Services Series 6 and 9.)
2 CERES. Medical Research and You. Questions for research subjects to ask. *Bull Med Ethics* 1991; **67**: 4.
3 Sackett D L, Haynes R B, Guyait G H, Tugwell P. *Clinical epidemiology: a basic science for clinical medicine*. Little, Brown, 1991.
4 Audit Commission. *Annual report*. London: HMSO, 1993.
5 Details of Ombudsman's report 1993, published July 1994.

Chapter 3
On risk in medicine

Robert Maxwell

Partner: THE KING'S FUND

Reading the popular press, listening to comment on the broadcast media, the citizen may be forgiven for believing that medicine can be a risk free activity. But all medical care is based on probabilities, and every act of diagnosis and treatment involves risk. Are the public and the patient helped to differentiate between relative and absolute risk? What is the difference between risk in terms of membership of a group, and individual risk? What part does an understanding of risk play in informed consent, and are we always sensitive to obtaining informed consent before doctors act? What is the implication of all this for litigation, and is there any way in which we can avoid the destructive role played by litigation in medical care abroad? What is the difference between a risk factor and an associated factor? What sort of language are we going to use in talking to the public, and to the individual patient, about risk?

Author:	Dr Robert Maxwell	*Chief executive, King's Fund*
Convenor:	Professor Marshall Marinker	
Members:	Ms Annabel Feriman	*Journalist*
	Professor George Freeman	*Department of General Practice, Charing Cross Hospital Medical School*
	Mr Peter Griffiths	*Director, King's Fund College*
	Dr Anthony Hopkins	*Director of Research Unit, Royal College of Physicians*
	Dr Jeffrey Roberts	*Medical Defence Union*
	Professor Ian Russell	*Research and Development Director, NHS Wales*
	Professor Nicholas Wald	*Chairman, Wolfson Institute for Preventive Medicine*
	Professor Albert Weale	*Professor of Government, University of Essex*

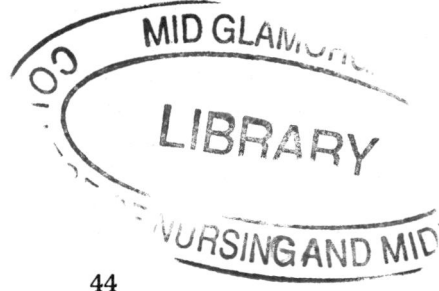

Introduction

By risk we mean a hazard or danger to patients and, more specifically, the chance of an unfavourable outcome for them. Risk is inherent in much medical treatment since treatment involves the use of potent interventions that have side effects which are unlikely to be free from hazard. A balance has to be struck between potential good and potential harm. In general this balance can be difficult to summarise and is not well communicated to patients. Indeed its nature is often not well understood by healthcare professionals. The purpose of this chapter is to explore how risks to patients can be better understood and better communicated, and what can be done to reduce them.

Obviously patients have no monopoly of risk. Professionals are also exposed to a variety of risks, as are managers, healthcare institutions and medical suppliers. Nevertheless the focus in this chapter will be on the risks run by patients. There is a story by Gerald Durrell about a boy, Adrian, who is left an elephant in his uncle's will.[1] Adrian has no idea what he is going to do with this bequest. He asks his friend Mr Puckelhammer for advice. The latter has none to offer. "Stop fretting yourself," he says, "we'll think of something." "It's all very well for you to keep soothing me," Adrian replies, "but I'm the one that's got the elephant." In terms of who bears the risks in medical care it is, in the end, the patient who has the elephant.

Interwined with the topic of risk in medicine is uncertainty,[2] but the two are not the same. Whereas in conditions of uncertainty we may have little or no idea of the implications of taking one course of action rather than another, the notion of risk implies that we know something about the balance of probabilities between good and bad effects. Without such knowledge medicine would have no claim to be a science. Much medical treatment involves some measurable probability of harm as well as some measurable probability of benefit. The probability of a particular harm can be expressed mathematically, as a continuous variable between zero and one, representing the proportion of adverse occurrences in a large number of individuals placed in similar circumstances.[3] This does not specify what the outcome will be for any particular individual, for whom the occurrence will either happen or not. It summarises the experience of patients on average. Generally, the risk of an unfavourable outcome for any individual will depend not on a single variable but on the interplay of several.

Risk can be thought of in absolute or relative terms. At times the latter is clearer than the former, for example "It is ten times more likely that this will happen to you than that will happen." Nevertheless, when the outcomes include chances of death or major harm, it is important to grasp both the relative and the absolute risks involved in the various treatment options, including that of doing nothing. Indeed, communicating relative risk can be misleading without at the same time anchoring it in the order of magnitude of the absolute risk.

Often the risk benefit profile of particular procedures, drugs or other therapies is not known reliably. Scientific research has to be carried out involving a large number of cases, observing what may be rare but substantial side effects and assessing long term outcomes. Such research is neither easy nor cheap. Yet the case for more of it, of good quality, is overwhelming. Medical history shows many examples of the extensive practice of therapies that ultimately have turned out to bring no benefit and to have put patients at risk of harm. It would be silly to assume that this cannot happen now, bearing in mind quite recent examples of unforeseen side effects, the wide variations in clinical practice, and the extent to which the majority of medical care still lacks rigorous scientific assessment of its effects on sufficiently large numbers of patients to be statistically reliable.

Physicians and risk

The practice of medicine calls for a wide range of qualities and skills—for example hands, heart, and head; compassion and toughness; willingness to listen and ability to explain; self confidence and self criticism. Among those that are not easily combined are, on the one hand, focus on the individual and, on the other, the ability to think statistically. Clinicians need a better understanding of risk and uncertainty than most of them have, both in a general sense (the nature of risk) and in particular instances (the statistical chances of specific therapeutic side effects and the associated variables).

Accurate quantification of risk usually requires large databases, which may have to be continually updated. In conditions of complexity and variation, it may well be that the human brain simply cannot hold and analyse all the relevant information without assistance. In any case, why not make the task easier? Hence the case for clinical guidelines, not to replace the best judgment of the clinician concerned but to provide a disciplined framework for it. Hence also the need for easy access by the individual clinician to an accurate database, preferably in the interactive questioning mode that computer systems can offer. It is also essential that the databases are compiled and maintained with the highest standards of intellectual honesty and rigour.[4]

It has been asserted that clinical autonomy is dead.[5] This is not the case. Nor has the fundamental justification for it changed, which always ought to have been an advantage to the patient. What has changed is that there is far more evidence than ever before about risks and variation in outcomes, and the responsible physician needs to bring that evidence to bear in exercising clinical judgment.

Patients and risk

Extraordinary as it may seem, patients in England still have no clear right to know the risks they face in treatment. The standard is still basically the Bolam test[6]—any physician has to justify what he or she did by reference to a body of responsible medical opinion. This applies to the communication of information, as to other aspects of treatment. Thus whether to inform or not is in English law less a matter of patients' rights than of physicians' duties, the latter being defined by custom and practice, rather than by any objective standard or principle.

Nevertheless the law shifts and Lord Scarman's opinion in the Sidaway case[7] points the direction of movement. (This was a case in which Mrs Sidaway was left disabled and in pain following a rare complication of spinal surgery. There was a dispute as to whether or not she had been advised of the complication. Apart from this dispute about the facts, there was also dispute about the law. Had she not been informed, then Lord Scarman would have differed from his colleagues in the standard to be applied. He would not have relied on the Bolam test.) It will not be long

---

An example of balancing pros and cons

Try explaining this to a patient who has had a transient ischaemic attack, and who has a carotid stenosis of 75%

Continue with medical treatment:

Stroke risk is 17% in next year

Have operation now:

Run risk of stroke of 7.5% in next 30 days, but if you avoid this, your risk in the next 11 months is 2.8%

---

before the test moves more towards what a reasonable patient would wish to know—and a good thing too.

That would not mean that every physician must force every patient (however unwilling) to know the risks (however remote) that they face. Some patients make it quite clear that they do not want to know. Others may be in a state of mind in which it is manifestly unkind to thrust information on them.[8] Most will need time and support to absorb information about serious risks, and to balance the pros and cons of different options (see box). Physicians have a duty (within the constraints of current knowledge) to know the risks, but then their duty is to judge what to say and how to say it. The standard ought to be what a reasonable patient, in the situation which the actual patient is known by the doctor to be in, would want to know. Deviation from this standard can properly be justified—but can only be justified—by the exercise of the physician's considered judgment based on the facts of the case and the patient's wishes, characteristics, and behaviour.

Risk can be associated with not providing (or advising on) a benefit, as well as arising from intervention. Examples might include the pros and cons of taking folic acid during pregnancy, or aspirin as a secondary prevention measure after an initial heart attack. There can thus be risks of omission as well as commission.

Patients should, in principle, not be exposed to risks when these are not justified in terms of a compensatory personal benefit from their treatment. The potential benefit of innovation to other patients would not justify imposing a risk on an individual that could not be justified by that individual's best interests. The case is no different in research—whether clinical or preventive—where there may be substantial uncertainty over the benefits. In such instances particular care is needed with explanation and consent. What happens, however, if patients want the treatment more quickly and under fewer controls than the state considers appropriate? New drugs for AIDS patients provide an instance of this dilemma. Inevitably, cost will be one consideration where the state has to pay attention to alternative uses for the money required. Nevertheless, it seems to us that more attention than in the past ought to be paid to the wishes of the patients concerned—individually and via patients' associations—at least on the issues of acceptable risk, if not on acceptable costs.

There is almost always an uneven balance of power between practitioner and patient. To some degree this can be redressed by increasing the quantity and quality of information available to individual patients, patients' associations and representatives, and the public at large. Physicians should wecome this. The argument that making risk explicit is confusing and frightening does not bear examination. Most members of the general public can understand the concept of risk and respond logically to survey questions that ask them to put a value on avoiding specified risks.[9] This should not surprise us. After all, the quantification of risk is similar to the assessment of odds, which is familiar enough to anyone placing a bet or doing the pools. Moreover, risk is basic to many other aspects of life—transport choices, for example.

Communication of risk

It is my belief that many physicians are inadequately prepared to communicate risks clearly yet sensitively, despite repeated calls from the General Medical Council to develop this aspect of medical education, and most patients are unprepared to receive this information as an integral part of their medical treatment.

Risks are perceived differently according to how they are conveyed. The difference between 98% and 99% probability of survival sounds small, but it is actually a halving of the risk of death! If two alternative treatments are offered, of equal effectiveness and risk, the alternative presented in terms of higher survival rate will be consistently preferred, by patients and doctors alike.[10] The manner of presentation of risk can therefore be important.

Quantifying the size and nature of the risk that ought to be conveyed is not easy. Nor are some of the assumptions transferable across national or cultural boundaries. For example, loss of a testicle is "worth" ten times as much in the Irish courts as in the UK (G J Roberts, Medical Defence Union, personal communication).

Patients need time to absorb and reflect on information. Interactive video can provide a useful tool for this purpose. Video programmes are now available on a range of common conditions for which there are genuine choices of treatment, based on different preferences in risks and benefits.[11] Interestingly, many patients seem well able to absorb this information and use it. They turn out to be more risk-averse to surgery than their surgeons.[12]

Too often the processes for obtaining written consent are perfunctory in the extreme, and trivialise what is being done. The objective becomes to obtain a signature rather than (as it should be) to record a considered choice. "Usual warning given" in the notes, or "UWG" for short, ought not to be an acceptable record that risks have been properly discussed with the patient. Furthermore, the courts have made it clear that it is the reality of the consent rather than its form which concerns the law (for example, Chatterton v Gerson). Obviously, signatures should not be the issue. Indeed obtaining a signature can be coercive and is often done, one suspects, more to protect the interests of the professional or the institution than in the interests of the patient.

There is some evidence, albeit limited, that time spent communicating may also be cost effective. For example GPs who spend longer explaining, prescribe less.[13] Of course that might not imply cause and effect. But three randomised controlled trials of the links between communication and outcome, for patients with chronic conditions, indicated that patients who asserted themselves more in their conversations with their doctors, and who showed more emotion (particularly negative emotion) and elicited more information, had better health outcomes.[14]

Overall there is a long way to go to raise communication of risk to even a passable level. But communication is by itself not enough. It has to be based on reliable information, and on clearer concepts of risk than most physicians and patients now have. Concepts of risk can be effectively communicated by diagrams, for example by using graph paper and shading in black an appropriate proportion of squares to indicate the likelihood of adverse occurrences.[9]

Reducing risks

Biases and errors are sometimes programmed into systems (as in the Birmingham pathology cases) and will occur unless the systems are changed. This argues for the regular review of systems, as an important institutional discipline.

Some therapeutic risks are unavoidable because of variations in outcome. Nevertheless, risk can be reduced by the way in which a service or institution is run. Patients have the right to assume that those who care for them are competent, exercise due care, and minimise risks. While the occurrence of negligence is low, it happens in about 1% of acute, non-psychiatric cases.[15] Everything possible ought to be done to eliminate it, even if this means contravening loyalty to colleagues or to the institution. Similarly, patients ought to be able to assume that the hospitals and other medical institutions that they use are so organised and managed that they are not exposed to avoidable risks. As Florence Nightingale wrote, it is the first requirement of a hospital to do the sick no harm.[16] If we are honest, there is a long way to go before patients can be confident that all the institutions that make up the NHS—or for that matter the private sector—have taken all reasonable measures to protect their safety. Medical audit[17] and management,[18] and institutional accreditation (E Scrivens, unpublished report) are all aimed at making our institutions safer.

There is also a duty on the part of doctors, nurses, and other healthcare professionals to protect patients from any colleague whose practice is for some reason unsafe. Too often loyalty to colleagues and cumbersome procedures have inhibited people from taking action.[19] The signs are that this will change, and so it should. Any doctor or nurse who allows a colleague to put patients at risk of serious harm is failing in his or her own professional duty.

What duty, on the other hand, do patients and the public owe their doctors? It seems reasonable that we should be expected to use services responsibly—not, for example, making night calls that are frivolous.[20] Do we also have a duty to behave in ways that do not put our health at unnecessary risk? In principle, I think that we do, but personally we do not accept the right of a clinician to withhold treatment from someone on the grounds that their conduct makes them unworthy. Once we take that route, none of us deserves treatment since none is likely to be wholly blameless in terms of health behaviour. Smokers are easy to pick out, but weight, exercise, alcohol, diet, risk-taking in leisure pursuits . . . where would we stop? Moreover, since behaviour has a variable impact on health status, interrelating with genetic factors, we

---

Conclusions and recommendations

- Physicians have a duty to understand the risks of adverse outcomes from the treatments that they prescribe or undertake; they should have the relevant information and should review it whenever the risks for any individual patient are substantial and serious. They should discuss these risks with the patient, unless they take a considered decision not to do so for reasons that are in the patient's best interest

- This often implies access to large databases. Access via computer on an interactive basis, so that physicians (and sometimes patients) can interrogate the relevant database, can be helpful. So can clinical guidelines

- English law is shifting to the basis indicated by Lord Scarman in his minority speech in the Sidaway case.[7] It will become a presumption that patients should be given the information that a reasonable person would want in order to make up his or her mind about the treatment options that are available. The patient's expectation will become more important than it has been, while the physician's duty will remain. There will be a better balance between the two. Such a change is long overdue.

- Clinicians need training to understand risks and to communicate them; the signs are that many patients understand risk quite well if properly explained[9]

- Patients have a legitimate right to assume that those who treat them are competent, that they will exercise due care and that they will minimise the risks of treatment; they also have a legitimate right to assume that the institutions in which care is delivered are as safe as competent management can make them

- While the main responsibility for high standards of care lies with the providers (professions and institutions) there is also an opportunity for purchasers to use their influence to protect patients, for example by writing into contracts good risk-management procedures and acceptable standards of explanation

---

would end up by penalising those who are poorly endowed genetically. Trying to explain to people the health risks that they run through their behaviour, and trying to help them alter it, is another matter.

References

1 Durrell G. *Rosy is my relative*. London: Fortuna Paperbacks, 1969.
2 O'Brien B. *What are my chances, Doctor? A review of clinical risks*. London: Office of Health Economics, 1986.
3 *Risk: analysis, perception and management*. London: Royal Society Study Group, 1992.
4 Freemantle N, Maynard A. Something rotten in the state of clinical and economic evaluations? *Health Economics* 1994; **3**: 63–7.
5 Hampton JR. The end of clinical freedom. *BMJ* 1983; **287**: 1237–8.
6 Bolam v Friern Hospital Management Committee [1957], 2 All ER 188, 1 WLR 582.
7 Sidaway v Governors of Bethlem Royal Hospital [1985], 1 All ER 643.
8 Tobias JS, Souhami RL. Fully informed consent can be needlessly cruel. *BMJ* 1993; **307**: 1199–201.
9 Philips PR, Russell T, Jones-Lee MW. *The empirical results of individual valuation of safety: results of a national sample survey in the economics of safety and physical risk*, Oxford: Basil Blackwell, 1989.
10 McNeil BJ *et al*. On the elicitation of preferences for alternative therapies. *N Engl J Med* 1982; **306**: 1259–62.
11 Kasper JF *et al*. Developing shared decision-making programs to improve the quality of health care. *Quality Rev Bull* **18(6)**.
12 Barry MJ, Mulley AG, Fowler FJ, Wenneberg JW. Watchful waiting vs immediate transurethral resection for symptomatic prostatism: the importance of patients' preferences. *JAMA* 1988; **259**: 3010–17.
13 Audit Commission. *A prescription for improvement: towards more rational prescribing in general practice*. London: HMSO, 1994.
14 Kaplan SH, Greenfield S, Ware JE. Impact of the doctor-patient relationship on the outcomes of chronic disease In: Stewart M, Roter D, editors. *Communicating with medical patients*. Newbury Park, Sage Publications.
15 Brennan TA, Leape LL, Laird NM, *et al*. Incidence of adverse events and negligence in hospitalised patients. Results of the Harvard medical practice study 1. *N Engl J Med* **324(6)**: 370–6.
16 Nightingale F. *Notes on hospitals*. 3rd Ed. Longman Green, 1863.
17 Hoffenberg R. *Clinical freedom*. Nuffield Provincial Hospitals Trust, 1987.
18 Youngberg BJ, editor. *Essentials of Hospital Risk Management*. Gaithersburg, MD: Aspen, 1990.
19 Stacey M. *Regulating British medicine: The General Medical Council*. Chichester: John Wiley and Sons, 1992.
20 Beecham L. Night calls should be limited to genuine emergencies say GPs. *BMJ* 1994; **308**: 1387–8.

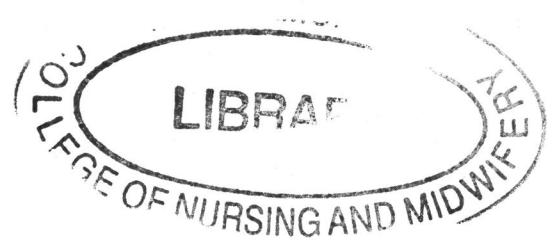

Chapter 4
How should health policy be modified by the evidence of medical practice variations?

Klim McPherson

Partner: NATIONAL ASSOCIATION OF HEALTH AUTHORITIES AND TRUSTS

Medical practice variation is a characteristic of almost every aspect of health care—the provision of resources, the processes of care, and the outcomes. Much of the current thrust in standard setting and quality assurance seeks to reduce this variation, in the name of better quality. What is most salient about this variation is that it is rarely if ever correlated with variations in demography and morbidity. Rather it is the vagaries of policies, technological beliefs, and idiosyncratic human behaviour that we see as reflected in the data. With so much uncertainty around, how can we plan health care rationally? What are the dangers of standardising, of becoming prematurely concrete in our thinking? Do medical practice variations compound human error, or reduce its impact?

Author:	Professor Klim McPherson	*Professor of Public Health, University of London*
Convenor	Professor Marshall Marinker	
Members:	Dr Helen Clayson	*General Practitioner, Cumbria*
	Mr Peter Coe	*General Manager, East London and City Health Authority*
	Mr John Cooper	*Chief Executive, Royal Free NHS Trust*
	Professor Roger Higgs	*Professor of General Practice, King's College London*
	Professor Jack Howell	*Professor of Medicine, University of Southampton*
	Mr Philip Hunt	*Director, NAHAT*
	Professor Ray Robinson	*Professor of Health Economics, University of Southampton*
	Dr Morton Warner	*Executive Director, Welsh Health Planning Forum*

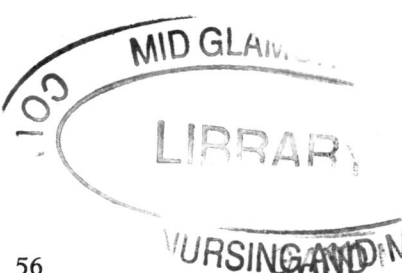

Introduction

Without doubt the politics affecting health care planning would change if the true implications of medical practice variations (MPV) were more widely appreciated and understood. Health policy would inevitably be different. This chapter sets out to describe the nature and scope of these variations and problems of their interpretation as well as the pitfalls that could result from ignoring or misunderstanding them. It ends with some of the challenges to the major stakeholders in health care policy that are consequent to an informed view of MPV. We take MPV to include all activities in health care, not just those which may be designated as medical.

The existence of MPV and their broad extent have been known for around 20 years.[1] Indeed the initial work of Glover[2] in the 1930s, demonstrating large difference in the prevalence of tonsillectomy among school children, began the realisation that for some of the health care provided its relationship with need was obscure. In the time since then the true nature and causes of much of the variation have been further consolidated, at least in aggregate.[3] This work demonstrates that the tonsillectomy example is not atypical and unusual, and that systematic and persistent variations exist between countries and between small geographical areas in the incidence of expensive and possibly risky treatments. These variations are the rule and not the exception, and they relate to individual decisions being made in good faith for the benefit of individual patients, which are mostly consistent with sound medical practice.[4] Medical practice variations represent, therefore, clear evidence for an important lack of consensus about the appropriateness of much health care provision.

Yet the impact this knowledge has had on health policy as such is small. For example, ministers and pundits are still heard to claim that the more patients admitted, the better, as if all treatment was necessarily equally beneficial or sufficiently cost-effective. Since, in general, MPV only usually provide evidence of a lack of consensus, the extrapolation to policy is not necessarily straightforward.[5] In the internal market, for example, MPV provide little useful guidance about the appropriate amount of care to purchase because quantity is rarely a reliable guide to quality. What they do is provide some comparison of quantity of care relative to that of other communities, and thus they can be used to benchmark notions of appropriateness.

In this chapter we will concentrate on the implications of MPV for current health policy. We must interpret this rather broadly as encompassing policy not only for the organisation and delivery of health care itself but also for research priorities and for the appropriate involvement of citizens in the delivery of that health care. One of the major reasons for the apparent failure of any obvious and useful connection between MPV and health policy is the lack of understanding of the particular relevance of MPV to that policy.

What are the relevant boundaries of health policy?

In addressing the question of the policy implications of MPV, the nature and limitations of health policy itself need to be considered. A policy is a general statement of principle and/or objectives which governs action. Public policy is such a statement on behalf of government or a government agency (or in a democracy an aspirant for government). Health policy refers to public policy for the health of the population and for the appropriate interventions of government in the provision of health care services. Fundamentals of public policy are often not stated as such, but may be imputed from lower order statements of policy and systematic patterns of action by public agencies.

Some elements of public policy in health are very long standing, others more recent. We suggest that there are three fundamentals of health policy, the first two of which are very long standing:

- To promote the health and wellbeing of the population. Today this traditional objective is expressed in the health gain objective
- To protect the citizen from avoidable harm
- To promote the autonomy of the free citizen through availability of choice and respect for consumer preference. This is an important and growing emphasis of policy in the latter decades of this century—that is, much more recently than the first two. A main objective of policy in recent years has been to empower consumers *vis-à-vis* providers.

> ### Fundamentals of health policy
>
> - Promote all aspects of the health of the population
> - Protect citizens from avoidable harm
> - Promote autonomy of free citizens to enjoy their own health

Why are MPV important for health policy?

We will take MPV primarily to be systematic (that is, non-random) variations in standardised rates for particular treatments, or important aspects of treatment, at some sensible level of population aggregation.[6] This may include referral rates from primary to secondary care or from secondary care itself.[7] These variations are usually observed between countries, regions, districts, specialists or GPs, and the implications of the particular MPV depend on the level of population aggregation. Clearly MPV measured between regions are likely to have different causes than those between GPs, and hence the implications in terms of cause as well as of effect will be very different.

Then one needs exhaustively to question how plausible an artefactual explanation—to do with data collection or recording—is in creating apparent variations. Once the MPV are thus legitimately designated as such, the policy issue then depends on how important these variations might be for attributable variations in outcome and in costs.

Thus long standing differences between standardised surgical rates for benign conditions have often been observed between countries of Europe, and particularly between North America and Europe, and these are often taken to be a reflection of differences in wealth and in incentive structures in the healthcare system.[8] Because they are understood in the context of other differences in culture and lifestyle, the pertinence of such contrasts may be ignored. However, equally large systematic differences are observed between neighbouring districts in a single country or region. In this situation, they might implicitly be attributed to small numbers or to minor idiosyncrasies of particular areas.

The importance and policy relevance of MPV would then depend on how far these can be correlated with relevant morbidity rates, and most research indicates that this correlation is rarely significant.[9] Almost all attempts to explain MPV by concomitant variations in relevant disease or need rates have failed. Much more commonly variation is seen to be associated with supply variables of various kinds. Most often, individual clinical decisions or practice styles can best explain variations in care between small areas of health provision. However, the main point of comparing small areas is quite simply that often the only major differences in aggregate characteristics are the particular health professionals making the decisions.[10]

The research strongly suggests that most common medical and surgical interventions do vary systematically between neighbouring small areas. The amount of variation is a function of the kind of intervention and not particularly of the country where the observations are being made.[11] The systematic variation for some things, like the treatment for benign prostate disease, is much more variable than, for example, treatment for acute appendicitis. Hysterectomy, for instance, is highly variable between countries,[12] but it is also highly variable around the national average within countries. Thus it was estimated in 1986 that while around £42 million was spent on hysterectomy, this would rise to £130 million if current US hysterectomy rates were applied to England and Wales.[6] Moreover, the variation observed between district health authorities, of around twofold, classifies hysterectomy as a moderately discretionary operation.[13] It is likely, however, that more than 80% of hospital admissions exhibit more variation than this.[5] Cholecystectomy, on the other hand, is much less variable between neighbouring hospital areas than is hysterectomy, but it is none the less highly variable between countries. This suggests that there is a strong consensus for cholecystectomy in each country, which is different from country to country, since all attempts to find intrinsic national differences in need have failed.[14]

For some important parts of medical care, systematic variations do not exist and this is a crucial part of the understanding; best

---

Why are MPV important for health policy?

- MPV are common
- Most MPV are large and systematic
- MPV have considerable implications for cost and outcomes

estimates suggest that around 10% of hospital admissions constitute care that is determined largely by unambiguous medical need. Some interventions vary with morbidity rates and there is no (or very little) discretion or uncertainty associated with treatment choices. Other interventions vary enormously but the consequences may be benign from a policy standpoint, because the cost and outcome variations are minimal.

Sources of MPV

An epidemiological perspective

The epidemiological research into MPV, where they exist, is able to distinguish in principle between three distinct causes of systematic variation. Mostly these variations relate not to irreversible treatment choices but rather to a threshold. The questions concern the knowledge about outcomes associated with treatment options at particular levels of disability, symptoms, or stage, and it is here that these variations are important.

- They may be largely a manifestation of *clinical uncertainty*, in circumstances, which are common when the relevant research into outcomes simply has not been done with sufficient rigour. This may be because to do so would be extremely difficult, but it also may be because assumptions are made without empirical legitimacy. Thus wide variation in treatment choices can remain perfectly consistent with medical knowledge.
- They may be manifestation of *clinical ignorance* of research that might indicate alternative treatment strategies and hence result in more homogeneity. This happens if dissemination of research and its implications lags well behind rigorous research itself or if research simply is not understood or believed.
- They may be manifestation of genuine *informed preferences* that

---

Major sources of MPV

- Clinical uncertainties
- Ignorance of relevant research
- Individual informed preferences

---

give rise to variations in treatment which respect those preferences in full understanding of their attributable outcome.

Each of these putative causes has important and different policy implications. The bulk of the literature points towards the first as being easily the most important. However, the kind of uncertainty being held responsible is not necessarily acknowledged explicitly; indeed, it is sometimes vehemently denied. Thus uncertainties are referred to as implied uncertainties where the practitioners may not acknowledge actual uncertainty. The distinction made here between uncertainty and ignorance is that the former is manifested by practice styles uninformed by scientific evidence yet to be obtained. Often they are necessarily based on hunch, scientific extrapolation, hope, personal experience, and so on. Ignorance is taken here to mean the decisions that are taken where the empirical or theoretical scientific evidence that already exists is ignored or forgotten, and is possibly never understood or even studied. The assumption is that such knowledge would alter practice styles, were it known.

The tools of medical research have produced staggeringly impressive results but there remain staggeringly impressive uncertainties. The relationship between the pursuit of clinical science and the pursuit of clinical practice is complicated.[14a] The objectives of the former are to establish the best clinical response to particular circumstances while those of the latter are to respond to a particular patient, which might often override the obligation to search for the truth. This latter action imperative tends to be strongly and vicariously imposed on managers, policy makers, and politicians.

A health professional perspective

The classical doctor-patient interaction is such that a patient relies on a doctor (or health advisor) to advise and sometimes to decide on the most appropriate treatment for the condition being investigated. In this relationship the above distinctions are absolutely central because a patient wishing to express his or her preference will in general rely on the doctor for information.[15] In this process, expressed uncertainties are disconcerting for an ill patient. They are disconcerting particularly because a patient cannot easily distinguish between ignorance and uncertainty in his or her advisor. Expressed uncertainty will have varying degrees of genuine legitimacy which might well remain opaque to a patient, who may then wonder whether another advisor would be (or appear to be) less uncertain. This is a major reason why expressed uncertainty is disparaged at most levels of medical encounter.

Differences between the response of individual doctors will occur because of differences in their experience, personalities, motivation, and values. There are also differences in their knowledge and skills and, related to this, their self confidence. Further, their environments will differ: the structure and organisation of the teams within which they work, and their relationships with colleagues and provider units.

Clinical knowledge may be perceived as collections of facts or truths, which comprise the dominant medical view. This can give rise to an awareness or anxiety that one knows only a small proportion of what can be known and may sometimes lead to lack of confidence and uncertainty, and this may result in some intellectual dishonesty. Today's medical facts may often be no more than current hypotheses, liable to be disproved and modified by new evidence.

In using NHS resources for investigation and treatment, the doctor will be influenced by his or her own knowledge of outcomes and perception of which outcomes are desirable. This may well raise conflict between two ethical principles—the primary responsibility to the patient on the one hand, and the responsibility to the community to use resources efficiently and effectively on the other. How much the doctor will seek to understand the utilities and the preferences of the patient and then how much that will influence the clinical choices will be a complicated balance.

Response to the existence of MPV

Medical practice variations seem therefore to suggest the existence of formidable problems for which the solution is varied, often somewhat obscure and possibly vague, and tends to have no particular or obvious policy implications. Hence it is not surprising that the response can often be inappropriate. However, there is little doubt that much of the current initiative in the research community for outcome assessment has been instigated by persistent observation of unexplained variations.[16]

> ## Responses to uncertainties
> - By patients
> - By policy makers
> - By health care givers

That MPV are largely concerned with genuine uncertainties is central to making the connection between MPV and policy in the broader health provision community. It is this thesis which most people have the greatest problem with. There is evidence for a ubiquitous reluctance to countenance the true extent of medical uncertainties concerning appropriate medical pratice—among potential consumers, among policy makers, and among the caring professions.

The reasons for this must be related to a legitimate desire to diminish the importance of the threat of disease, on the part of the ill citizen, and to emphasise the professional and scientific role of medicine, on the part of the professionals. Policy makers have an ambiguous relationship with both, which is interesting. They neither want to diminish the importance of disease nor necessarily to exaggerate the professional role of carers, but none the less they are equally reluctant to acknowledge the true extent of uncertainties in medicine, because this likewise would diminish the importance of the enterprise they are concerned with.

Most importantly, to perceive the true extent of uncertainty itself requires a formidable body of knowledge and understanding, usually invested in health professionals alone. Policy makers must perforce take their cues from the informed practitioner, who is unlikely to emphasise his or her own true uncertainties, for the reason expressed above.

Because of this, several kinds of inappropriate responses may occur. There is, for example, an implicit tendency to believe that for population-based treatment rates appropriate provision will lie somewhere between the two observed extreme rates, where variation exists. This can be observed in several studies[17, 18] of the monitoring of changing rates when they have been publicised, and of course has no absolute justification whatsoever. Among the total context of all variations observed, the mid point in one region may well be completely extreme in another. To import the mid point intervention rate from the USA to here might well involve a doubling of the UK's health expenditures.[19] To export ours to the developing world is obviously completely out of the question.[20]

Thus planners and economists tend to see variation as an opportunity for savings, where possibly uniformity seems to be against the nature of the biological process being observed. The question that is raised is what should be considered "normal biological limits", as in blood pressure? Without assiduous study of variations the extent of need-related variations are grossly exaggerated.[21] Planners and economists tend to assume that the distribution shold be shifted towards the lower resource use end of the observed continuum. However, where medical intervention rates are low, as in the UK, normative standards often suggest that higher rates of intervention are more appropriate, for example in coronary artery bypass grafting or renal dialysis. Medical care is dynamic. A level of variation is often seen as a necessary reflection of a normal process of diffusion of innovation. But it is not at all clear that proper mechanisms exist to enable anybody to learn from the existence, extent, and nature of varations.[22]

Another response is to imagine that appropriate indications for intervention exist and that decisions should be subjected to guidelines to ensure more uniformity and consistency. Again, the basis of this response will depend on the true extent of uncertainty and on the true opportunities for genuine informed preferences. There is a tendency to promote guidelines based to some degree on unevaluated average practice styles, where no obvious explanation can be found for practice style differences. The problem here will be the need to include all possible beneficiaries and hence apply universal criteria that may not be individually beneficial nor result in a preferred legitimate option.

A proper response is:

- To identify the true areas of clinical uncertainty and, giving due respect to their importance and existing research, set about assessing the effectiveness of available treatments.[16]
- To ensure that information is disseminated to enable practitioners to keep up with such research
- To offer patients opportunities for informed choices.

To enable this to happen it is essential for planners and purchasers to recognise which aspect of health care provision is determined by certainty, and with what degree of ignorance of efficient preferences related to knowledge of outcome.[23]

Barriers to the appropriate modification of policy

With respect to the three objectives of policy outlined above, clearly the determinants of MPV have different implications: MPV generally are only indirectly, though importantly, relevant to the first objective of promoting wellbeing. On the other hand, where they are a manifestation of ignorance or uncertainty, they are directly relevant to the second, and where MPV reflect genuine uncertainties, increasing the role of consumer choice under that uncertainty should be an important object of policy.

In this context there are several important relevant issues to do with medical information which are crucial. The first is clinical freedom and its role in rational health policy.[24] In the burgeoning activity of the introduction of clinical guidelines, the role of individual professional judgment is being eroded and the implied threat to the importance of clinical judgment is clear. Partly as a consequence, only certain kinds of clinical uncertainties can be readily acknowledged without being threatening. These are usually concerned with new treatments, for which uncertainty is thus legitimised.

The important point here is that uncertainty can be confused with ignorance too readily, and if genuine uncertainty is taken as a manifestation of ignorance, then it is unlikely to be readily acknowledged. This is particularly true in the dominant medical paradigm of scientific truth and certainty. To be able to admit to uncertainty often thus requires an unassailable authority itself, which most professionals would be reluctant to claim. Unevaluated but well established (often very common) treatments present particular problems in this context.

Thus the existence of large and systematic MPV for common treatments can be taken as evidence of implied uncertainties which may not be acknowledged as manifestations of real uncertainty by the profession. The incentive to evaluate the relationship of practice style with outcome is then compromised, in spite of indirect evidence for considerable uncertainty. This is important, as we shall see, when randomised trials are the only method of attributing cause to effect. Randomisation is only deemed to be ethical when clinicians are genuinely, and individually, uncertain.

On the other hand, the placebo effect of medical certainty may be real, is mostly unmeasured, but may be very important therapeutically. Therapeutic efficacy may itself thus be compromised by frank admission of uncertainty. There is an increasing body of evidence which demonstrates, for instance, that patients who adhere to treatments do better even if the treatment is a placebo in a double blind trial.[25, 26] In most cases assiduous adjustment for putative confounding factors makes little difference to this comparison. There are perfectly sensible biological mechanisms for such effects, but as yet they have been poorly investigated.[27, 28]

Thirdly, the role of consumers in decision making is important, since providers have the responsibility for decision making under uncertainty where consumers may have the dominant preferences. The policy question is therefore to examine which is the most important and how consumers can become appropriately involved, in a cost-effective manner.

Affecting actual policy among decision makers

Once the causes of MPV and their interpretations are established, policies for changing practice on the basis of research evidence should be implemented. To be able to do this, it is first of all necessary to establish who are the different parties with a stake in medical practice decisions. These will include *inter alia* individual clinicians, professional organisations, district purchasers, GPs, and patients. Beyond this, it is necessary to establish the multiple determinants of their behaviour, including the general social, professional, and organisational structures within which they work and the incentives—implicit and explicit—to which they react. This approach recognises that addressing MPV is not simply a case of disseminating information on best practice and expecting a rational response in terms of, say, clinical behaviour. Rather, it highlights the multiple objectives and constraints (some of them perverse and conflicting) to which any individual or organisation can be expected to respond.

A couple of examples might illustrate these points. District

health authorities now have responsibilities as purchasers of health care. Variation between providers in terms of, say, length of inpatient stays, repeat outpatient appointments, and day surgery rates should all be of relevance to purchasers because they influence the volume of care (and its outcomes?) that can be purchased from given budgets. As such, it might well be appropriate for the NHS Management Executive to monitor purchasers' performance in terms of the services they secure as far as these "performance indicators" are concerned. However, such an approach needs to be based on appreciation that district health authorities are presently judged on a whole range of indicators, some of which have only tangential (and uncertain) relevance to the maximisation of health gain. We need to address the issue of how MPVs and their management can be given a higher profile in the context of priority overload.

GP fundholding, for example, offers a limited example of the ways in which incentives can be used in this respect. GP control over budgets might lead to more rational and cost-effective prescribing, but this needs to be evaluated with respect to outcome. There is also some evidence that fundholding has addressed problems such as tardy pathology laboratory performance and unnecessary repeat outpatient attendances. Perhaps there is a general lesson here: the devolution of power in decision making, alongside the financial responsibility for these decisions, including a share in the gains and losses, might be mechanisms that we wish to consider in more detail.

Another set of policies governs expenditures on health care. With public monies, policy will be directly concerned firstly with economy—it is always the object of policy to minimise public expenditure as far as is consistent with achievement of the public purpose. Where expenditures vary substantially because of MPV then there is a requirement of public accountability to justify the expenditures, in the context of manifest (and acknowledged) uncertainties about benefit.

Effectiveness is, and should increasingly become, a dominant concern where choices have to made against limited budgets—it is a general requirement of accountability for public expenditures to demonstrate that monies have been expended effectively. Medical practice variations are relevant where they suggest the possibility of ineffective expenditures. Ignorance must be the main target, once it is identified.

MPV and health policy

- Where they arise from ignorance: to protect from harm and to promote effectiveness of public expenditures

- Where they arise from uncertainty: in health policy there must be a presumption in favour of minimising public expenditures, by choosing the cheaper intervention, until the marginal benefit of higher rates can be justified

- To promote the role of informed preference and consumer autonomy; it should be noted that this principle may well sometimes conflict with the previous one

Thirdly, equity is an ever present criterion; even under governments that readily accept inequalities in distribution of private incomes, it is accepted as responsible policy that public expenditures on health should benefit citizens equitably. Medical practical variations suggest inequity, except where they are obviously a legitimate manifestation of efficient choices.[29]

This analysis suggests that for health policy the main interests of MPV are threefold (see box).

It is not a part of health or other public policy to promote everything that may be a good thing but to pursue defined and specific purposes appropriate to the role of government in a liberal democratic society. Public and health policy is also constrained by its instruments. The question has to be not only whether this is an appropriate end of policy but also are there any means available to government, or that can be invented within the constitution, to allow it to do anything about it?[30]

What are the policy implications for the future?

We are left with three strong assertions which ought to give rise to policies and priorities that take account of the above. Firstly, the existence and extent of MPV indicate that standards of care are generally not based on adequate knowledge of outcomes.[31] This is because the necessary assessments have not been done to establish the correct biological or medical theory. Such assessments need not be randomised controlled trials but they do have to be methodologically rigorous.[32] Secondly, there is ample evidence that research findings do not find their way into clinical practice as readily as they might. Thirdly, mechanisms for enabling patients to choose treatments in accordance with the real uncertainties and their own preferences are, as yet, poorly developed.[33] Where standards of care could be based on adequate knowledge of outcome and are not, then appropriate information dissemination and professional and consumer involvement must be a high priority.[34]

Uncertainties are well protected in the current healthcare delivery system, sometimes possibly for sound therapeutic, social, and economic reasons, but the research into precisely how and when this protection is appropriate is poorly developed. Further study should lead to an assessment programme that takes on board the prioritisation of relevant outcome research, which is currently being developed and which is adequately funded. Such an assessment programme must choose areas to investigate which are common, expensive, exhibit important (implied) uncertainties, represent real treatment choices, and are amenable to rigorous assessment.

Then it will be important to investigate assiduously the likely attributable outcomes and their probabilities from the literature or databases, if necessary. Where significant uncertainties remained, then randomised trials would be indicated and hopefully these would be funded.[35] Where necessary, the extent of patients' expectations and experience should be evaluated and assessed. Information packages that are designed for decision makers, to bring them up to date with current research where required, should be assessed. This could include packages for health professionals or for patients.

Crude decision analysis can also be extremely illuminating, particularly when combined with sensitivity analysis.[36] These investigations may indicate outcome studies to be essential, and in this context it is important to acknowledge that MPV themselves offer ethical options for assessment which are very rarely adequately exploited.[37]

Although much medical practice remains unevaluated, many examples exist of where knowledge is available but is not put into practice. Many North American foundations supporting research have recognised this problem for the last decade. Now, research and development bodies within the UK are giving dissemination and development much more serious attention.

In the purchaser/provider world, especially with the growth of

GP fundholding, how the fundholders and other purchasers can be come well informed about what works and what doesn't is important. Financial and other incentives may well take knowledge through to a change in practice. The opportunities for such a mechanism to be exploited are underdeveloped. All this depends on adequate and specific information systems being in place to monitor outcomes.

In pursuing these objectives, the need for homogeneity for its own sake is pointless. Medical practice often varies legitimately, because of well-founded differences of opinion. Medicine is not an exact science, and in many respects is not a science at all, only science based. Legitimate and useful responses to MPV include: formal clinical protocols for evaluation and then standard setting, as well as deliberate measures to diffuse proven innovations more rapidly. Perhaps there is also a need to focus on outliers, to encourage review and assessment of practice by clinicians.

Identification of barriers to "normal" practice which can be removed by management action is important. For example, if less complex procedures are routinely placed at the end of operating lists, they cannot be done as day cases. This is quite common.

In terms of medical education, the right balance between certainty and uncertainty, between what is known and what is believed, should be explicitly considered. Attempts to standardise to a dominant paradigm by the selection of students and curriculum may be counterproductive. There is no evidence that the General Medical Council's new curriculum recognises this requirement as such—it simply describes the need to teach principles without indicating what this means.

The challenges are to implement the provision of care in such a way that, where possible, the assessment of the effects of treatment on quality of life and functioning from the patient's point of view is, or can be, routine. Secondly, the challenge is to create a decision making process that is capable of maximising the appropriate opportunities for using all the available data about patient outcomes. In this process, understanding the limitations of these data are just as important as the knowledge they provide.

The evidence for common uncertainties in clinical practice is overwhelming and clearly important. Carving away at key parts of them is the dominant component of the outcome research agenda.

Policy implications of MPV

- Illegitimate certainties are no basis for health policy
- Investment in dissemination of research findings
- Prioritised outcome evaluation programmes
- Information systems enabling more routine outcome assessment
- Evaluation of the extent and the role of uncertainty in medicine
- Enhancement of appropriate opportunities for enabling patients to exercise choice in decision making

However we have sought to draw attention to some of the potential problems in priority setting and in the evaluation of treatments, where consumer input is important and possibly neglected. These considerations are important methodologically as well as substantively, and their methodological implications are poorly investigated as yet. In the end, illegitimate certainties provide no basis for rational health policy.

The acceptability of greater patient involvement in decision making is essentially unevaluated. The role of this involvement on outcome remains untouched. Randomised trials deny choice and yet they are the means toward the final arbiter of effectiveness. It is possible that by reducing choice the effectiveness of therapies in unblinds trial is thus attenuated. More comparison of preference trials and randomised trials is required.[33]

Although it is important to evaluate the effectiveness of medical interventions, it is well recognised that even a spurious belief in the unproven effectiveness of interventions may enhance their value.

The true role of uncertainty in medicine has yet to be properly investigated and certainly understood. This state of affairs arises in part, of course, because uncertainty fits very uneasily into the dominant medical paradigm. If the evidence for it were properly accepted, what happens in medical school would change, much of what happens in clinical practice would have to change, much of what happens in media coverage of medicine would also change, and certainly what now happens in the evaluation of outcome would change.

References

1 Bunker JP. Surgical manpower: a comparison of operations and surgeons in the United States and in England and Wales (1970). *New Eng J Med* 1970; **282**: 135–44.

2 Glover JA. The incidence of tonsillectomy in school children. *Proc R Soc Med* 1938; **xxxi**: 1219–36.

3 Anderson TV, Mooney G. *The challenges of medical practice variations.* London: Macmillan Press, 1990.

4 Chassin M R, *et al.* Does inappropriate use explain geographic variations in the use of health care services? *JAMA* 1987; **258**: 2533–7.

5 Wennberg JE, McPherson K, Caper P. Will payment based on diagnostic related groups control hospital costs? *N Engl J Med* 1984; **311**: 295–300.

6 McPherson K. *Variations in hospitalisation rates: why and how to study them.* London: King's Fund Institute, 1988.

7 Coulter A, Seagroatt V, McPherson K. The relationship between general practice outpatient referral rates of elective admissions to hospital. *BMJ* 1990; **301**: 273–6.

8 McPherson K, *et al.* Regional variations in the use of common surgical procedures: within and between England and Wales, Canada and the United States of America. *Soc Sci Med* 1981; **15A**: 273–88.

9 Wennberg JE. Population illness rates do not explain population hospitalization rates. *Med Care* 1987; **25**: 349–9.

10 Wennberg JE, Gittlesohn A. Small area variations in health care delivery. *Science* 1975; **182**: 1102–8.

11 McPherson K, Wennberg JE, Hovind OB, Clifford P. Small area variations in the use of common surgical procedures: an international comparison of New England, England and Norway. *N Engl J Med* 1982; **307**: 1310–4.

12 McPherson K. Why do variations occur? In: Anderson TF, Mooney G, editors. *The Challenges of medical practice variations.* London: Macmillan Press, 1989.

13 Coulter A, McPherson K. The hysterectomy debate. *J Soc Affairs* 1986; **2**(4): 379–96.

14 McPherson K, *et al.* Do cholecystectomy rates correlate with geographic variations in the prevalance of gallstones? *J Epidemiol Community Health* 1985; **39**(2): 179–82.

15 Wennberg JE, Barnes BA, Zubkoff M. Professional uncertainty and the problem of supplier induced demand. *Soc Sci Med* 1982; **16**: 811–24.

16 Wennberg JE. What is outcomes research? In: Gelijns AC, editor. *Medical innovations at the crossroads.* Vol 1. *Modern methods of clinical investigation.* Washington DC: National Academy Press, 1990: 33–46.

17 Dyck FJ, Murphy FA, *et al.* Effects of surveillance on the number of hysterectomies in the Province of Saskatchewan. *N Engl J Med* 1977; **296**: 1326–9.

18 Wennberg JE Blowers L Parker R, *et al.* Changes in tonsillectomy rates associated with feedback and review. *Pediatrics* 1977; **59**: 821–6.

19 Aaron HJ, Schartz WB. *The painful prescription, rationing hospital care.* Washington DC: Brookings Institute, 1984.

20 World Bank. Feacham RGA, Kjellstrom T, Murray CJL, *et al,* editors. *The health of adults in the developing world.* Oxford: OUP, 1992.

21 Morgan M, Mays N, Holland WH. Can hospital use be a measure of need for health care? *J Epidemiol Community Health* 1987; **41**: 269–74.

22 Wennberg J. Which rate is right? *New Engl J Med* 1986; **314**: 310–11.

23 Caper P. Variations in medical practice: implications for health policy. *Health Affairs* 1984; **3**: 110–19.

24 Hoffenberg R. *Clinical freedom.* London: Nuffield Provincial Hospitals Trust, 1987.

25 Coronary Drug Project Research Group. Influence of adherence to treatment and response of cholesterol on mortality in the coronary drug project. *N Engl J Med* 1980; **30**: 1038–41.

26 Horowitz RI, Viscolli CM, Berkman L, *et al.* Treatment adherence and risk of death after myocardial infarction. *Lancet* 1990; **336**: 542–5.

27 Wolf S. Effects of suggestion and conditioning on the action of chemical agents in human subjects—the pharmacology of placebos. *J. Clin Invest* 1950; **29**: 100–9.

28 Philips DP, Todd RE, Wagner LM. Psychology and survival. *Lancet* 1993; **342**: 1142–5.

29 Wennberg JE, Freeman JL, Culp WJ. Are hospital services rationed in New Haven or over utilised in Boston? *Lancet* 1987: 1185–8.

30 Evan RG. The dog in the night time: medical practice variations and health policy. In:

Anderson TF, Mooney G, editors. *The challenges of medical practice variations.* London: Macmillan Press, 1990.

31 Cochrane AL. *Effectiveness and efficiency. Random reflections on health services.* London: Nuffield Provincial Hospital Trust, 1972.

32 Anonymous. Databases for health care outcomes. *Lancet* 1989; **335**: 195–6.

33 McPherson K. The best and the enemy of the good: randomised controlled trials, uncertainty, and assessing the role of patient choice in medical decision making. The Cochrane Lecture. *J Epidemiol Community Health* 1994; **48**: 6–15.

34 Kasper JP, Mulley AG, Wennberg JE. Developing shared decision making programmes to improve quality of health care. Quality review bulletin. *J Quality Improvement* 1992;**18**: 182–90.

35 Roos, *et al.* Therapies for benign prostatic hyperplasia. *JAMA* 1992; **268**: 1269–70.

36 Barry MJ, Mulley AG, Fowler FJ, Wennberg JE. Watchful waiting vs immediate transurethral resection of the prostate for symptomatic prostatism. *JAMA* 1988: **259**: 3010–17.

37 Wennberg J, Roos N, Sola L, Schori A, Jaffe R. Use of Calim's data systems to evaluate health care outcomes: mortality and reoperation following prostatectomy. *JAMA* 1987; **257**: 933–6.

Chapter 5
Medical advances and the future of old age

Raymond Tallis

Partner: AGE CONCERN

Traditionally, geriatricians have made much of the fact that old people are not necessarily exhibiting the symptoms of the aging process but actually suffer from diseases, many of which can be treated. Conversely, disease processes may be seen as manifestations of aging cells, organs or systems. The insights of evolutionary gerontology suggest that many of the genes which are thought to be associated with disease (those that predispose man to diabetes, hypertension, obesity, cancers, and so on) fail to be eliminated by natural selection in the early development of man, because of an investment in reproduction rather than repair. This suggests that the boundary between reversible and irreversible aspects of decline in old age may not be immutable. What are the perspectives of geriatricians, general physicians, gerontologists, sociologists, and economists?

Author:	Professor Raymond Tallis	*Professor of Geriatric Medicine, University of Manchester*
Convenor:	Professor Marshall Marinker	
Members:	Dr Edward Dickinson	*Senior Lecturer, Royal College of Physicians*
	Dr Iona Heath	*General Practitioner, London*
	Professor Tom Kirkwood	*Professor of Gerontology, University of Manchester*
	Dr Peter Mayer	*Director, Clinical Services for the Elderly, Selly Oak Hospital*
	Professor Graham Mulley	*Consultant Physician, St James', University of Leeds*
	Dr Michael Rowe	*Consultant Geriatrician, Bath*
	Professor Anthea Tinker	*Professor of Social Gerontology, University of London*

Health care in old age: an agenda for discussion

The provision of adequate and appropriate health care for older people is the greatest challenge facing health services in developed countries. There is widespread fear that increasing numbers of people carrying a progressively heavier burden of disease and disability will "swamp" acute services and consume an increasing proportion of even an expanding health budget. There are already signs of panic, with ill-judged attempts by managers to ration health care according to age, despite expert opinion that this is not only morally dubious but also clinically irrational.[1]

Beyond specific health economic issues there are wider economic issues. Can the nation (it is asked) afford to support growing numbers of increasingly disabled older people? Economic considerations may be disguised as concerns about the appropriateness of "intensive", "invasive", "hi-tech" health care for very old and often frail individuals. The (unsurprising) observation that individuals utilise the greatest amount of health resources in the last year of life prompts the question whether treatment of very sick old people tends to follow the law of diminishing returns or, worse, brings modest increases in longevity at a disproportionate cost in discomfort. Repeatedly, one hears it said that adding life to years is more important than adding years to life, that it is the quality not the duration of life that matters and that "care and comfort" may be a more appropriate goal than "cure", even though, as Grimley Evans has pointed out,[2] curing is also a form of "caring". And it is often asserted that there is more to be gained from other approaches

---

An agenda for discussion

- What are the consequences of a successful assault on the major disabling conditions of old age?

- Will individuals die of "old age", understood as something separate from disease?

- Is it better to die from the former than the latter?

- Will aging, too, be "treatable"? If so, what do we hope to achieve?

- What, ultimately are the ends and aims of medicine?

---

than medicine narrowly construed: prevention and health promotion; improving social conditions; and education.

Even if one accepts the central role of traditional medical treatment and also takes an optimistic view of likely medical advances—that they will lead to increased life expectancy without increased disability—unanswered questions still remain, and these provide the agenda for this chapter.

Anxieties abut the future health care of older people

It may be safely assumed that the next few decades will witness an aging of the elderly population.[3] Will this increased longevity be bought at the cost of more prolonged morbidity and disability? The relevant literature is rich in argument and suppositon but relatively poor in empirical data of the right kind. There is plenty of evidence—from surveys in the United Kingdom[4], the United States,[5] and elsewhere—that the prevalence of chronic illness rises sharply as one moves from younger old age to older old age. Disability is a more powerful determinant of consumption of health and social care responses than illness *per se*, and here the trends seem to be alarming, with an exponential relationship between age and the prevalence of disability,[6] reflecting the strong association between age and chronic cardiovascular, musculoskeletal, and neurological diseases, and the global and potentially chronic impact of even focal, acute illnesses in the biologically aged.[7]

Increased need cannot be offset by diminished health expectations; on the contrary, there is evidence that these are rising amongst old people.[8] Younger old people expect more than the nonagenarians whose views were sampled in *Life after ninety*.[9] Succeeding cohorts will be less willing to accept inadequate health and social services. Even before the recent reforms, satisfaction with the NHS was falling.[10]

Does increasing longevity inevitably mean increasing need? Notional futures of old age, set out in figure 1, range from the blackly pessimistic to the wildly optimistic. The first curve is a diagrammatic presentation of the current situation in which Mr or Mrs Average remains essentially free of disability until, say, 60 years of age and then incurs an increasing and accelerating burden of disability until he/she dies at the unisex average of, let us say,

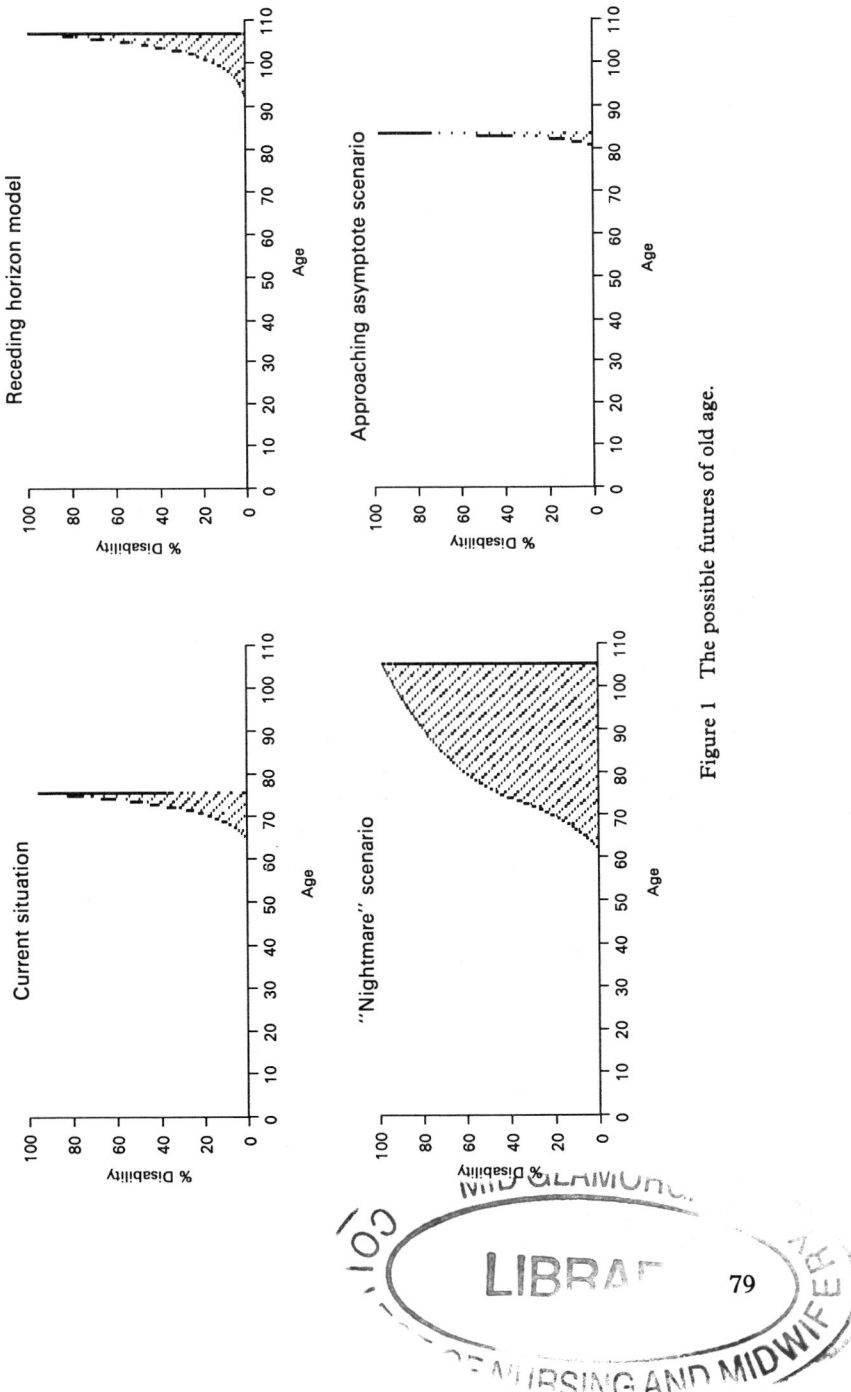

Figure 1   The possible futures of old age.

75 years of age. (This example, of course, takes no account of enormous variation between individuals, of the uneven progress of disability, of premature death in youth and middle age, of sudden death in old age, etc.) The area to the right of the curve may be thought of as representing person-years of impaired, disabled, handicapped, or in some way medically unsatisfactory existence. There are three possible developments:

1 *In the receding horizon model* the onset and progress of disability is postponed to precisely the same extent as death itself. The number of years of disabled existence remains unchanged
2 *In the "nightmare" scenario* the onset and progress of disability is as at present, but death is postponed. This corresponds to the grim scenario of Gruenberg[11] and Kramer[12] in which there is a "pandemic of mental disorders and associated chronic diseases and disabilities"
3 *In the approaching asymptote scenario* both disability and death are postponed, but the former more than the latter, so that the interval between the onset of disability and death is reduced ("compression of morbidity").

Option 3 is, for many, the ideal; it was initially postulated by Fries[13] and has been widely discussed, often critically, since. Fries' idea is linked to that of death from old age—a relatively painless and disability-free affair arising out of "homoeostenosis"—and progressive approximation of the "health span" to the life span.

Available data do not permit us to determine which way things are going. The general household survey reveals that, although there has been an increase in the proportion of people of all ages reporting a long standing illness (suggesting probably a lowered threshold for pronouncing oneself ill), the upward slope is flattest in the oldest. In the last two decades, the percentage of the overall population reporting long standing illness has increased from 21 to 34%, while for the over-75s it has increased from 62 to 69%— proportionately much less.[4] There is also encouraging recent information from the national long term care surveys in the USA,[14] based upon Medicare files, which represent over 97% of the elderly population. They record a decline in the total prevalence of chronically disabled community dwelling and institutionalised elderly people, for all of the three age strata (65–74, 75–84, and 85+). The proportion of non-disabled persons who became

---

Anxieties about the future health care of older people

- The trend has been towards an exponential relationship between aging and the presence of disability

- Health expectations are rising among older people

- The nature of the future relationship between longevity and disability is uncertain

- Recent UK data indicate that the trend to increased reporting of long standing illness is *less* in the over-75s

- Recent US data show increased life expectancy to be associated with a *decline* in age-specific disability

---

disabled after 2 and 5 years was also significantly lower in the later than the earlier time interval. These changes remained significant after mortality and age adjustment. Increases in life expectancy above 65 were associated with declines in the age-specific prevalence of chronic disability,[15] as well as mortality improvements for disabled persons. The jury, however, is still out.

Medical advances

Projecting health care for the future on the basis of demographic trends and current levels of morbidity in older people does not take into account possible medical advances. These may be divided into better use of existing treatments and new treatments. Although what follows focuses on the latter, the former may have major beneficial impacts. For example, avoiding inappropriate prescribing could reduce adverse drug reactions by up to 50%[16] and more universal provision of good conventional diabetic care could dramatically reduce long term morbidity.[17]

Rheumatological problems

Major progress may be expected in joint disease. Surgical advances will result from the use of new materials for prostheses, new approaches such as arthroscopic re-lining and re-shaping of joints,[18] and improvements in less well developed prostheses (elbow, shoulder, ankle, etc). Better perioperative care will mean that more frail elderly people will be able to undergo operations.

81

We may expect analgesics with improved risk–benefit ratios. Better prevention of secondary adverse effects, including muscle wasting, joint deformity, and disability, seem likely. Finally, less empirical treatments, based upon clearer understanding of the biochemical mechanisms of degeneration and inflammation are probable.[19] Control of the current epidemic of osteoporosis and related fractures, with more global use of preventive strategies— diet, exercise, reduction of alcohol and smoking, hormone replacement therapy—and earlier and better treatment of more precisely diagnosed osteoporosis may be anticipated.[20]

Neurological problems

The major neurological problems are stroke, non-vascular dementia, and Parkinson's disease. Advances in the prevention of stroke (mainly coming from wider application of knowledge of risks factors and their modification),[21] in the limitation of the damage arising out of stroke (in particular the cascade of events following an ischaemic insult),[22] and in novel methods of reversing neurological impairments,[23] may be anticipated. People with non-vascular dementias will benefit from a better understanding of the relevant molecular genetics,[24] from the identification of markers and diagnostic tests, permitting earlier diagnosis and treatments before damage has become widespread and irreversible, and from better drug therapies.[25] Earlier diagnosis on the basis of objective markers will also permit treatment of Parkinson's disease when the damage is still focal, its effects are less complex, and neuroprotection is not too late.[26] Subtyping cases according to more precisely defined aetiologies will enable treatments to be less empirical.[27]

Blindness and deafness

Reduction of blindness due to glaucoma, cataract, and diabetic retinopathy seems likely. It is reasonable to anticipate better treatments of these conditions and of senile maculopathy, based upon increased understanding of mechanisms. For example, cataract prevention by enhancing dietary intake of antioxidants seems a distinct possibility.[28] Similar improvements in deafness seem less likely, though important gains will be made with more user-friendly hearing aids and better understanding of why people with hearing impairments so often either do not have or use aids.

Areas in which it is expected that morbidity can be reduced

- Joint disease and osteoporosis
- Neurological problems: stroke, non-vascular dementia, and Parkinson's disease
- Blindness
- Deafness
- Additionally, with the introduction of techniques to reduce invasiveness, surgery will become more available to frail, old people

---

Surgery

Surgery is undergoing the most rapid evolution in its history, with a shift from knife-based conventional surgery to "keyhole" and orifice surgery, using fibreoptic endoscopy for diagnosis and treatment.[29] This, combined with better promotion of wound healing and improved understanding and control of the physiological sequelae of operations,[30] will improve the safety of surgical options for frail old people.

Overview

Most of the feasible medical advances seem likely to make a disproportionate impact on disabling conditions—such as arthritis and stroke—rather than life threatening ones, and one might expect their net effect to be to reduce, rather than increase or merely postpone, chronic morbidity and disability. We may therefore hear less rather than more about the "the failures of success".[11] This will be enhanced by a gradual shift towards medical care being a "partnership of experts" between patient and doctor, so that the former will make an informed choice. The increase in the number and user-friendliness of health information sources for elderly people will contribute to this process and to improving general health.[31, 32]

Aging and disease

With more effective ways of retarding the onset of diseases and limiting their adverse effects, will "old age" come to play a bigger role in limiting the quality and duration of life? The notion that old age will take over where disease leave off assumes that the two are distinct. This is not self evident. Could not "aging" merely be the sum of subclinical disease processes that have not advanced far enough to assume the distinctive features of ICD-categorisable decay? This suggestion is more complex than it might initially appear. First, subclinical disease likely to be mistaken for aging would need to be multiple to have sufficient cumulative impact, and one could argue that the vulnerability necessary to fall victim to a multiplicity of diseases is due to aging. Alternatively, low levels of disease might cause visible deterioration or death only in an organism that had been brought near to the threshold by other changes—presumably those of aging. Less disturbance is required for a pathological process to produce dysfunction and, because of "homoeostenosis", disturbances, displacements from the normal range, are more likely to be irreversible.[13] Thirdly, a disease is subclinical only so long as it has not been recognised by a clinician. Clinician recognition depends upon observation of characteristic features: subclinicality may be maintained to a high level of damage by age-related failure of the body to produce characteristic (usually adaptive) responses, modifying the presentation of disease, so that it may present as non-specific decline.[7] If aging is characterised by de-differentiation of disease, and the narrowing repertoire of disease manifestations expressed in the predominance of the "geriatric giants" (falls, immobility, confusion, and incontinence), we could postulate a point of convergence of aging and disease, where disease elicits no specific features; alternatively, we could argue that aging is disease that, due to the failure of adaptive responses, elicits no specific features.

These conceptual difficulties in demarcating aging from disease are compounded by the empirical ones. At present, there are few symptoms and signs that fully meet the criteria for a "true" aging process—one that occurred universally in old age and only in old age. Conditions that seem to meet that criterion are often trivial (and scarcely life threatening), such as wrinkling of the skin, or developmental, such as the menopause, which has only incidental dysfunctional consequences. Some significant and serious pathology comes close to universality—for example, senile maculopathy, osteoarthritis, prostatic hypertrophy—but no one is going to suggest that these can be dismissed as "mere" aging with its implication of a lack of therapeutic activity. The uncertainty surrounding the characteristics of the aging process—if it exists—in part reflects the methodological problem of defining study populations in order to identify "pure" or "physiological" aging.[33] Moreover, there is often no sharp demarcation between changes that are typically attributed to age and those that are given a diagnostic label; for example, the pathological changes seen in Alzheimer dementia are also seen in normal brains, the difference being only one of distribution and quantity[34] (though this may change when more robust genetic markers are identified).

There are obvious clinical, didactic, and (perhaps) political reasons for saying, with perhaps more confidence than the facts and concepts justify, that aging should be distinguished from disease. For disease is traditionally something that requires a therapeutic response; whereas, so far, aging is something that patients, carers, clinicians, and politicians feel no obligation to do anything about. Older people are at risk of being treated not as individuals but as points on a negative regression curve mapping "inexorable" decline in function.[35]

Even supposing aging and disease were clearly separable, they would still interact and converge, having a common ultimate outcome—death—and a common pathway to that outcome—homoeostatic failure. Would death by aging be an advance over death by clearly defined disease? Death in old age will seem more appropriate (or less inappropriate) than death in youth; and death from old age may be less unpleasant, not being associated with intrusive symptoms such as pain, nausea, shortness of breath, and gross disability. Instead, we may envisage a subtle and progressive reduction in "life space" associated with an increased probability of a death that is more easily achieved—as if the distance to be traversed between life and death is abbreviated. The image of death by aging as the end result of gradual but harmonious failure of all organs is attractive.[36] It is compatible with current conceptions of aging, which "lead to a picture in which there is progressive, roughly synchronous decline in function of many different organs." [37]

Aging approached from the point of view of a wary clinician afraid of missing a treatable condition is more elusive than aging approached from the standpoint of a biologist. No one looking at the different, highly stereotyped life spans of organisms could doubt that aging is something real and genetically determined. It is difficult to claim that it is only through hard luck or bad mouse-husbandry that experimental mice do not become centenarians.

According to contemporary evolutionary ideas, aging is a consequence of the neglect of repair mechanisms in favour of reproduction.[38] This is clinically attractive because it challenges the assumption that aging is an inevitable consequence of complexity, the "inescapable" wear and tear of any highly ordered system in accordance with the second law of thermo-dynamics. Wear and tear can be dealt with by repair; and this raises the possibility of intervention or reversal by mobilising or enhancing existing biological repair mechanisms. Numerous mechanisms for this "progressive, generalised impairment of function resulting in a loss of adaptive response to stress and in a growing risk of age-related disease"[38] have been postulated. Animal evidence suggests a polygenic basis for longevity, which would indicate that there is unlikely to be a single mechanism.[39] However, there may be a predominant mechanism. Alternatively, there may be an interaction between mechanisms so that intervention to reverse or prevent one mechanism may produce major benefits out of proportion to the separate contribution of that mechanism to the final aging process.[40] Threshold phenomena may be very important here. After all, the simple expediency of calorie restriction may produce significant gains in life span of rodents.

It is not inconceivable, therefore, that we may be able to slow down the aging process at some time in the future, though the effects of this in the long term may be difficult to predict; after all,

---

Aging and disease

- The distinction between aging and disease is not clear cut: they may converge, or aging may be a disease that has no specific features

- There are few symptoms and signs that meet the criteria for a true aging process

- Distinguishing between aging and disease is important because disease, which requires a therapeutic response, should not be dismissed as untreatable aging

- If predominant mechanisms among those involved in the aging process are identified, intervention to slow aging may eventually become possible, creating new dilemmas

---

the human organism is a very complex dynamic system and, for such systems, predicting the outcome of interventions is notoriously difficult.[41]

Aging, disease, and the ultimate aims of medicine[42]

Medicine has two aims, usually linked but sometimes in conflict: the relief of suffering due to disease and the prolongation of life. Probable advances in medicine will lead only to finite advances in life span, a palliation of transience rather than the achievement of immortality. This raises the question of what finite additions to a finite life span are worthwhile? When is the right time to die? According to Paul Valery,[43] it is when there has been

> total exhaustion of the possibilities of the system of an individual man. All the inner combinations of his capacities, incomplete in themselves, would be exhausted. He has told himself everything he knew.

We are a long way off that goal but it is reassuring to think that, contrary to popular opinion, increases in longevity are not inevitably going to be bought at the cost of increased personal suffering or an unacceptable pressure on the public purse. Managerial and political panic may not be the appropriate response either to hard-won medical advances or inescapable demographic trends.

References

1 *Ensuring equity and quality of care for elderly people. The interface between geriatric medicine and general (internal) medicine.* London: Royal College of Physicians, 1994.
2 Grimley Evans JG. Curing is also caring [editorial]. *Age Ageing* 1989; **18**: 217–8.
3 Office for Population Census and Statistics. *National population projections: 1992 based.* London: OPCS, 1994. (OPCS Monitor PP2 9411.)
4 Office for Population Census and Statistics. *The general household survey 1990.* London: HMSO, 1992.
5 Crimmins EM, Ingegnen DS. Changes in life expectancy and disability free life expectancy in the United States. *Popul Devel Rev* 1989; **15**: 235–67.
6 Office for Population Census and Statistics. *OPCS Surveys of disability in Great Britain, Report 1, the Prevalence of disability among adults.* London: HMSO, 1988.
7 Horan MA, Pendleton N. The boundary between ageing and disease. *Rev Clin Gerontol.* In press.
8 Abrams M. Third age lives in the next generation: changing attitudes and expectations. In: Warnes A, editor. *Human ageing and later life.* London: Edward Arnold, 1989.
9 Bury M, Holmes A. *Life after ninety.* London: Routledge, 1991.
10 Brook L. *Report for social and community planning research.* Bristol, 1992.
11 Gruenberg EM. The failures of success. *Milbank Memorial Fund Q/Health Soc* 1977; **33(1)**: 3–24.
12 Kramer M. The rising pandemic of mental disorders and associated chronic diseases and disabilities. *Acta Psychiatr Scand* 1982; **62** (suppl 285): 282–97.

13 Fries JF. Ageing, natural death, and the compression of morbidity. *N Engl J Med* 1980; **303**: 130–5.

14 Manton KG, Corder LS, Stallard E. Changes in the use of personal assistance and special equipment from 1982 to 1989: results from the 1982 and 1989 NLTCS. *Gerontologist* 1992; **33**: 168–76.

14a Sackett DL, Haynes RB, Guyait GH, Tugwell P. Clinical Epidemiology: a basic science for clinical medicine. Little, Brown, 1991.

15 Manton KG, Corder LS, Stallard E. Estimates of changes in chronic disability and institutional incidence and prevalence rates in the U.S. elderly populaton from the 1982, 1984, and 1989 national long term care survey. *J Gerontol* 1993; **48** (suppl): 153–66.

16 Lindley CM, Tully MP, Paramsothy V, Tallis RC. Inappropriate medication is major cause of adverse drug reactions in elderly patients. *Age Ageing* 1992; **21**: 294–300.

17 Kerr D, Haigh R, Intensive diabetes treatment: a new deal for old people? *Age Ageing* 1994; **23**: 89–90.

18 Dandy DJ. The present state of arthroscopy. *Minimally Invasive Ther* 1991; **1**: 51–6.

19 The process of inflammation. In: Maddison PJ, Isenberg DA. Woo P, Glass DN, editors. *Oxford Textbook of Rheumatology*, Vol 2, Section 3. Oxford: Oxford University Press, 1993; 285–360.

20 Grimley Evans J. The epidemiology of osteoporosis. *Rev Clin Gerontol* 1993; **3**: 13–29

21 Klag MJ, Whelton PK. The decline in stroke mortality. An epidemiologic perspective. *Ann Epidemiol* 1993; **3**: 571–5.

22 Sandercock P, Williams H. Medical treatment of acute ischaemic stroke. *Lancet* 1992; **339**: 537–9.

23 Tallis RC. Rehabilitation of the elderly in the twenty first century. *J R Coll Phys* 1992; **26(4)**: 413–22.

24 Mullan M, Crawford F. Genetic and molecular advances in Alzheimer's disease. *Trends Neurosci* 1993; **16**: 398–403,

25 Williams A. What will be new in neurology? *Update* 1993; 32–5.

26 Shultz CW Future perfect? Presymptomatic diagnosis, neural transplantation and trophic factors. *Neurol Clin* 1992; **10**: 567–93

27 Gibb WRG, Lees AJ. A comparison of clinical and pathological features of young- and old-onset Parkinson's disease. *Neurology* 1988; **38**: 1402–6.

28 Hankinson SE, Stampfer MJ, Sedon JM, *et al.* Nutrient intake and cataract extraction in women: a prospective study. *BMJ* 1992; **305**: 335–9.

29 Calne RY. OK Surgical technology. *BMJ* 1991; **301**: 1479–80.

30 Horan MA, Roberts NA, Barton RN, Little RA. Injury responses in old age. In: Evans JG, Williams TF, editors. *Oxford Textbook of Geriatric Medicine*. Oxford: Oxford University Press, 1992: 88–93.

31 Tinker A, McCreadie, C, Salvage A. *The information needs of older people: an exploratory study*. London: Age Concern Institute of Gerontology, King's College, 1993.

32 Rowe MJ, Tyler JS, Stephens N, Clarke J, Richardson K. An information centre for the elderly. *Care Elderly* 1991; **3**(1): 33–6.

33 Grimley Evans J. Ageing and disease. In: *Research and the ageing population*. Chichester: John Wiley, 1988. (Ciba Foundation Symposium 134.)

34 Hofman A, van Duijn CM, Rocca WA. Is Alzheimer's disease distinct from normal aging? *Lancet* 1988; ii: 226–7.

35 Maddox GL. Foreword: special issue on the Berlin ageing study. *Aging Soc* 1994; **13**: 475–82.

36 Toft AD. If I live to be a hundred . . . *Lancet* 1994; **343**: 434.

37 Kirkwood TBL How do risk factors for dementia relate to current theories on mechanisms of ageing? In: Huppert FA, Brayne C, O'Connor DW, editors. *Dementia and normal ageing*. Cambridge: Cambridge University Press, 1994: 230–43.

38 Kirkwood TBL. Biological origins of ageing. In: Evans JG, Williams TF, editors. *Oxford textbook of geriatric medicine*. Oxford: Oxford University Press, 1992: 35–40.

39 Martin GM. Biological Mechanisms of Ageing. In: Evans JG, Williams TF, editors. *Oxford textbook of geriatric medicine*. Oxford: Oxford University Press, 1992: 41–8.

40 Kirkwood TBL, Franceschi C. Is aging as complex as it would appear? *Ann NY Acad Sci* 1992; **663**: 412–17.

41 Gleick, J. *Chaos*. London: Cardinal, 1988.

42 Fox T. Purposes of medicine. *Lancet* 1965; ii: 801–5.

43 Valery P. *M. Teste*. New York: Bollingen/Pantheon: 99.

Chapter 6
Rational prescribing: How can it be judged?

Marshall Marinker
Philip Reilly

Partner: THE ROYAL COLLEGE OF GENERAL PRACTITIONERS

Everyone pays lip service to the goal of rational prescribing. Yet the term "rational" can be open to a number of interpretations. The "therapeutic conservatism" of the UK doctor is regarded by many scientists and managers in the pharmaceutical industry as a serious fault. Yet this conservatism has long been taught and encouraged by teachers of general practice.

Few aspects of medical process have been so subjected to analysis and attempted control, as prescribing by general practitioners. By and large there has been a belief that average prescribing rates and costs represent some sort of virtue, and higher quantities and cost must be critically examined. How can we balance the need to be parsimonious with resources in the NHS, to reduce iatrogenic damage, and at the same time to make available the most effective medications?

Authors:	Professor Marshall Marinker	
	Professor Philip Reilly	*Professor of General Practice, University of Belfast*
Members:	Ms Nicky Britten	*Lecturer in Medical Sociology, United Medical and Dental Schools of Guy's and St Thomas's*
	Mr Andrew Burr	*Pharmaceutical Adviser, West Glamorgan FHSA*
	Dr Gordon England	*Director, National Advisers' Support Centre*
	Professor Richard Hobbs	*Professor of General Practice, University of Birmingham*
	Dr Jaqueline Jollys	*Director of Research, Centre for Health Services Management, University of Nottingham*
	Dr Aly Rashid	*Course Organiser, University of Leicester*
	Mr David Taylor	*Health Economist, The Audit Commission*

90

Introduction

The term "rational" is much used in relation to prescribing. For example the Audit Commission's report *A prescription for improvement*[1] carries the subtitle *Towards more rational prescribing in general practice*. Rational, which means reasoned, is so often applied to prescribing, and so rarely to other clinical acts—diagnosis, investigations, hospitalisation, and so on—that one is driven to ask what special meaning attaches to the word rational in relation to prescribing. It is not difficult to detect the semantic overtone of "rationing", and indeed almost all of the literature on rational prescribing focuses on cost. Of course cost is most often referred to in relation to benefit, so that the aim of rational prescribing is expressed in terms of the efficiency of the care being provided.

Although we retained the term rational prescribing throughout the groundwork for this chapter, we were at pains in our earlier discussions to emphasise all the components of what might be described as a reasoned approach to prescribing, and not simply to focus on cost, or even efficiency, alone. The term "optimum prescribing" appealed to us. It is interesting that the Health Select Committee (see data from the Office of Health Economics in reference 1), which recently reported on prescribing, preferred the term "appropriate". By this they meant prescribing "which bases the choice of drug on its effectiveness, safety and convenience relative to other drugs or treatment (including surgery) and only takes cost into account when those criteria for choice have been satisfied."

This chapter will explore a number of issues, including the context in which prescribing is considered; prescribing as part of the clinical process; the problem of evidence; cost, risk, and benefit; managing for better prescribing; and future trends.

The context

Some 10% of NHS expenditure is accounted for by the cost of prescribing in general practice. In 1992/93 this amounted to some £3.55 billion in England and Wales. In 1978 some seven items per patient per year were prescribed; by 1992 this figure had risen to some nine items. By international comparison, the British patient is a relatively low consumer of medication, although international comparisons should always be read with caution because of the very varied social and welfare contexts in which the estimates are made. In 1990 the expenditure per British citizen was £64 compared with £91 in Germany, £107 in Italy, and £112 in France. Expenditure in Britain was about 23% below the Western European average.[2]

Quite apart from the prescribing choices that doctors make, a number of other factors contribute to inflate the volume and costs of prescribing:

- There is an increasing proportion of older people in the population; the expenditure on drugs for the oldest patients is up to 12 times that for the young
- One of the key intentions of the recent NHS changes is a shift of resources and activities from secondary to primary care; more conditions are therefore being treated by GPs, with the inevitable consequence that more drugs are prescribed in practice
- Moreover, the new contract for GPs encourages proactive care, case finding, and earlier diagnosis. More diagnosis leads to more prescribing
- The pharmaceutical industry, at the same time, introduces products intended for intervention earlier and earlier in disease processes. For decades, doctors have been encouraged to use drugs proactively. Oral contraceptives, hormone replacement therapy at the perimenopause, drugs to reduce moderate hypertension, cromoglycate in the prevention of atopic conditions, are all examples. More recently drugs have been introduced for the treatment of early benign prostatic hypertrophy. As new conditions or new therapeutic opportunities are defined, prescribing escalates.

All of these factors are self evidently contributors to improvements in health care. They seem to require only a rational prescribing response. However, there are also worrying data about prescribing that suggest deep irrationality:

- The range of prescribing levels in general practice is large and can in no way be explained by different levels of morbidity and demographic and socioeconomic factors. The Audit Commission gives the examples of hypnotics, anxiolytic, and lipid-lowering drugs. Harris has suggested that 40% of this variation in prescribing can only be accounted for by so-called "doctor factors"—the idiosyncratic choices which doctors make, independent of factors such as the social structure of their populations, the incidence and prevalence of disease, and so on (C Harris, personal communication)

- There is evidence that many important therapeutic substances are substantially underused.[3] Examples include failure to use inhaled steroids in asthma, ACE inhibitors in cardiac failure, and lytic therapy in acute myocardial infarction
- Some 3–5% of all hospital beds in the United Kingdom are occupied by patients suffering from adverse drug reactions.[4]

The response of the Department of Health to this very complex picture has by and large been limited to activities concerned with cost containment. Much of the profession's own literature on prescribing[5] has similarly urged a minimalist approach, a robust scepticism about innovations, the choice of generic alternatives, and the virtues of therapeutic conservatism. What different markers of quality prescribing would emerge from our discussions?

Little in the formal medical education of most doctors has prepared them for the task of prescribing. Medical students are taught pharmacology and applied therapeutics, but they are not taught about prescribing itself. They are not given the intellectual and interpersonal competences of constructing a therapeutic strategy: choosing between therapeutic alternatives and specific drugs; monitoring dose, progress, and compliance; negotiating the treatment with the patient, explaining risks and benefits; and managing the end point of therapy. The contrast between the relatively short time spent on these topics in medical education and the dominant role that prescribing plays in practice is remarkable.

Further, almost nothing is taught about the forces that shape prescribing: expert opinion; peer pressures; adult learning theory; marketing and sales techniques; patient expectation and demand; and budgetary controls. Some of this may appear formally during vocational training courses; much is left to the implicit and uncertain lessons of early practice.

Prescribing as part of a rational clinical process

One of our earliest conclusions was that we cannot look at rational prescribing in isolation from the rationality of the whole healthcare delivery system. Prescribing could be seen as the defining act of clinical intervention. In schematic terms it marks the end of the diagnostic phase, and the beginning of the therapeutic phase. Unfortunately, this seemingly elegant model ignores a number of irrational components in the clinical process. When the GP prescribes an antibiotic for a child with a cough, the diagnosis will probably be recorded as "bronchitis". However, bronchitis, in this case, is not so much the basis for the choice of drug but rather the alibi for it.

An analysis of the second national morbidity survey[6] suggests that variation between doctors in the levels of morbidity which they record is such that the differences can be explained only in terms of idiosyncratic choice of label, not in terms of real differences in morbidity. Similar findings emerged from a study of GPs reviewing video tape recordings of consultations with patients who presented with psychological symptoms.[7] The variance in the diagnoses made and the prescriptions that the doctors suggested was such as to suggest that the dominant factor in both diagnosis and treatment was the doctor's individual point of view.

The conclusion reached from the national morbidity survey study was that, since there was no firm link between the diagnoses selected by doctors and the true incidence and prevalence of morbidity in the patient populations, it would be unsafe to construct treatment protocols in general practice. This would only be true, however, if the starting point of protocols and guidelines was an established diagnosis without reference to minimal explicit criteria.

Doctors in the Western world, like their patients, are part of an instrumental culture. Action is valued above reflection. The pressures to diagnose and treat, even in the absence of a sound basis for action, are considerable. They can also pose substantial threats to the wellbeing of the patient. In a high proportion of consultations in general practice, the patient's problem cannot be formulated in terms of a disease process. In many such instances, therefore, the prescription is issued not as a response to a diagnosis but rather to signify the completion of the therapeutic encounter.

In order to put rational prescribing into the context of a rational clinical process, we identified five necessary components.

> ## The components of rational prescribing
> - A defensible formulation of the patient's problem
> - Clarity of therapeutic intention
> - Access to independent data on drugs
> - Communication with the patient
> - Follow up

A defensible formulation of the patient's problem

Patients consult because of symptoms rather than diseases. When a chronic or recurring condition has been established, the patient may experience exacerbations or changes in the pattern of symptoms. What characterises the work of the GP is what Balint[8] described as "the organisation of unorganised illness". The provenance of this organisation depends on a number of factors. The diagnosis may be formulated at the level of *symptoms* or at the level of *pathology*. Furthermore, the pathology may be supported either by physical findings and laboratory evidence, or it may be inferred from the history and the probabilities. A couple of examples illustrate the difference:

- The patient complains of recent heartburn but no other clue about the cause is forthcoming. The GP is likely to respond at the symptom level, and prescribe an alkaline mixture and a bland diet. The patient is instructed to return if the symptoms have not cleared within days.
- A diagnosis of duodenal ulcer with concomitant *Helicobacter pylori* infection can be arrived at only on the basis of investigation by gastroscopy, histology, and bacteriology. The response may well be a combined regimen of ulcer healing drugs and relevant antibiotics. The diagnosis and treatment rests on a more or less elaborated theory and picture of disease. In general practice, this is the exception rather than the rule.

The diagnostic roles of the GP and the specialist have been sharply contrasted.[9] The role of the specialist is to reduce uncertainty, to explore possibility, and to marginalise error. The role of the GP is to accept uncertainty, to explore probability, and to marginalise danger. When a 40-year-old obese woman complains that her legs swell in the middle of each month, the diagnosis may never proceed beyond the boundary between symptom and physiology. A small dose of thiazide diuretic may be prescribed in the attempt to relieve the swelling, although the condition (the rational basis for the prescription) would best be recorded as "swollen legs".

If the important probabilities have been explored, if the danger from a missed serious condition has been marginalised, then the level of uncertainty is acceptable and both the diagnosis and the treatment are rational. It is essential to add a caveat to this discussion of diagnosis, however. Because we are talking about medication, the emphasis has been on the physical component of the patient's illness. General practice is concerned with a holistic approach to the patient, valuing appropriately the physical, the psychological, and the social domains. The GPs prescription may therefore respond to social and psychological factors in the illness, and not only to the physical ones.

Clarity of therapeutic intentions

Treatment may be directed at:

- The relief of symptoms (as in the above example)
- The amelioration of the disease process (for example, the use of insulin in diabetes)
- The elimination of disease (by use of an antibiotic for an acute bacterial infection for example).

Unless the doctor is aware of the level of the diagnosis, it is unlikely that the therapeutic intentions will be clear. For this reason, rational prescribing must be seen in the context of rational diagnosis. A rational diagnosis is one that is defensible, one that can be confidently supported by evidence.

Diagnosis at the level of symptoms will be a common feature of good clinical practice in primary care. Sometimes, however, the prescription is not so much the response to an established diagnosis but rather the test of a hypothesis. For example, if the patient presents with non-specific lethargy but no other localising symptoms, a blood test may reveal a microcytic anaemia for which there seems to be no evident cause. The doctor makes a provisional diagnosis of iron deficiency and prescribes iron. The prescription may well resolve the problem, but it may do so not by correcting the anaemia. The response to treatment may illuminate the cause. If the patient does not respond to the iron, the GP will now need to look harder for the evidence of a hidden chronic disease, of which the anaemia is only the presenting facet. Clarity of therapeutic intention is contingent on a diagnosis made at an appropriate level of understanding.

Access to independent data

In chapter 1 some of the problems concerned with establishing the objectivity of data and the independence of the sources were rehearsed. It is arguable that no source can be totally disinterested. In terms of information about pharmaceutical substances, the different stakeholders, however scrupulous they are in collecting evidence and presenting it, must always be seen as being biased by their interests.

Leading specialists are properly involved in clinical trials around the time that new drugs are brought to the market, or when new indications are proposed for established products. They are then seen to be important endorsers of new therapies, and lecture widely about diagnosis and treatment—first to their specialist colleagues, and later, with their colleagues, to GPs. Of course their major motivation is the improvement of medical care. Nevertheless, they are also concerned with maintaining the relevance and importance of their own specialties, and they are concerned with their own reputations and the success of their own specialist departments and hospital trusts in an increasingly competitive internal market. The relationship between the pharmaceutical company and the endorsing specialist is therefore mutually supportive and beneficial. It must not be collusive.

Pharmaceutical companies, however idealistic their rhetoric and beneficent their support for medical education, research, and health and welfare projects, are also properly interested in their own commercial success. Inevitably the evidence that they will seek to emphasise will be that which supports these commercial interests.

The government, the Department of Health, and the health authorities are also biased. Although their public duty is to produce an efficient health service, it is recognised that they must do so within financial bounds. The task of government is not to provide the best possible health care for the least possible cost, but the best possible health care within a limited budget. However it is expressed in terms of efficiency, this task relies heavily on measures of cost containment.

There is clearly a gradient of self evident interest between, for example, a promotional video produced by a pharmaceutical company about one of its new products and an entry in the *British National Formulary*. One of the members of our group said that "of all the players, only the patients can be said to have legitimate interests." None the less, the biases of specialists, pharmaceutical companies, and government (and other stakeholders not here mentioned) are all legitimate. This legitimacy is, however, contingent on transparency—all research results, clinical opinions, and information on cost and benefit should be read with the interests of the providers of the information in mind.

Bias is only one of the problems in providing the GP with appropriate information about drugs. General practitioners are responsible for initiating treatment across virtually the whole range of clinical conditions, and for patients of all ages. It is therefore totally unrealistic to expect the individual GP to master information about some thousands of current medications available to NHS patients. Most individual GPs work with a personal formulary (rarely formalised) of some 300 drugs. The problem in composing group formularies is that each doctor's list of 300 is very different from that of all of his or her other colleagues.

The Audit Commission suggested the need for a framework into which information about drugs could be fed, so that the practitioner would be in a position to make informed choices. We suggest that such a framework might comprise nine components (see opposite).

Increasingly, cost-benefit analyses will include economic calculations that go beyond the immediate cost of a particular treatment or comparisons with alternatives. They will include the likely cost conseqeunces of the treatment on subsequent costs in other parts of the health and social welfare system. The patient's expected health gain, consequent on the treatment, should also be seen in terms of the relative costs of fitness and unfitness, employment and unemployment, and so on. The use of health economics in this way is still in its infancy. Given the financial constraints imposed on almost every healthcare system, it will grow.

A framework for information to facilitate rational prescribing

- Class, generic name, and proprietary names of drug
- Therapeutic actions
- Data about unwanted effects and interactions
- Indications and contraindications
- Recommended doses and regimes
- Costs
- Significant differences from previously established drugs in the same class, or drugs with an almost identical therapeutic intention
- A risk-benefit analysis
- A cost-benefit analysis

Communication with patients

Since patient autonomy is a key moral precept in clinical practice, the rationale of the prescription should be equally apparent to and accepted by doctor and patient. Such evident good intention is fraught with problems. The doctor's health beliefs are by and large informed by contemporary biomedical science. The doctor has a sense of likelihood based on epidemiological research, and of cause and effect based on laboratory and clinical experiment.

The widespread belief among members of the public that all sore throats should be treated with oral penicillin must, in the first place, have been created by doctors. None the less, the patient's health beliefs, although heavily influenced by those of the medical profession, are often quite differnt from the doctor's. For example, a patient who expects to be given penicillin because he has a sore throat will have his own views about cause, risk, and benefit ("Penicillin is a relatively safe and common drug, and it might help, and I am going on holiday tomorrow").

Different cultural groups have quite distinct beliefs about the origins of a variety of conditions, and they have their own lay terms to describe them. Beliefs about cause and treatment may be based on family tradition, on reading the popular press, on personality, and on much else. If the patient's beliefs are treated simply as inferior to the doctor's, the communication gap between doctor and patient will be unbridgeable.

The task of the doctor is to acknowledge the patient's belief, explore it, and incorporate both health beliefs into the patient's acceptance of the diagnosis, the treatment and the need for compliance. Not only will this require considerable interpersonal skills, it will require an extensive vocabulary of ideas in relation to risk and benefit—a topic discussed in chapter 3. It is important that the patient should understand the difference between *relative* risk ("If you take these tablets it will halve your risk of having a stroke") and *absolute* risk ("Your risk of getting a rash from these tablets is less than 1:10 000"). The significance of changes in relative risk will be much modified by the size of the absolute risk. However, these are statistical concepts, and may mean little to the patient. The patient may understand far better the notion of *analogous* risk ("Taking these tablets for the next 10 days is a lot less risky than driving your car over the same period"). Even when the doctor can explain notions of risk and benefit in analogous terms, there will still be the need to understand the *qualitative* nature of risk ("I would rather die from a stroke than survive damaged by it").

One of the most difficult tasks in an era of proactive medication, is the notion of deferred gratification. The doctor may invite a patient, who feels quite well, to take medication over many years, in the hope of avoiding or at least postponing a later catastrophic illness. If the patient experiences all too little gratification in his or her present life, the notion of deferred gratification will be quite foreign. Compliance is unlikely.

Even when these essential components of the patient's understanding have been addressed, there will be much else to convey: the timing of the medication, dose schedules, dietary advice, and so on. Ideally every prescription should be accompanied by a detailed set of information and instructions tailored to the unique situation of the patient being treated, written in language that the patient can understand. The average consultation time in British general practice is less than 10 minutes. Is it reasonable to expect the GP to be able to pay attention to all the elements of communication necessary to ensure that rational prescribing results in rational treatment?

Follow up

The vast majority of consultations in general practice are concerned with follow up. Even if the consultation is triggered by a new condition or event, the ethos of continuing care in British general practice, and the fact that the GP holds the unique central and continuing record of the patient's interaction with the medical profession, ensures this. In terms of prescribing, therefore, follow up will often be arranged in order to monitor the progress of the condition being treated, even if this is no more than a telephone call at the end of the week to ensure that the condition has resolved. For the majority of longer lasting conditions, however, there will be a need to monitor progress, the response to medication, required changes of dose or drug, and so on.

When the medication is long term, "repeat prescription" systems have been devised, and this has been greatly facilitated by the very rapid spread of information technology. These systems allow the practice to make some checks on compliance and to ensure the regular recall of patients for re-evaluation.

Because the care of patients with chronic conditions is increasingly being shared between general practice and specialist departments in the hospital, there is a growing need for interactive information systems between practices and hospitals. Without such interactive systems there will be a growing danger of duplication of medication, with consequent risk to health and life.

A footnote must be added, concerning the follow up of patients on long term medication. A seminal study[10] of patients on "repeat prescriptions" suggested that the patient's problem, and the therapeutic response to it, could be far better understood in terms of the patient's personality than in terms of morbidity and therapeutics. There are very many instances of patients on long term medication, where the diagnostic rationale is lost, obscure, or stated and untenable. The part that the drug plays in these very distinctive doctor-patient relationships is more complex than that of the well-documented placebo response. This study concluded with a rational explanation (in psychological terms) of a clinical situation that appears wildly irrational (in purely medical terms). In determining rational prescribing, the field of rational discourse must always be stated.

Key issues

The foregoing evidence and arguments suggest that judging the rationality of prescribing is a complex and often uncertain business. This is not a counsel of despair, however. As is so often the case, it is easier and safer to determine what constitutes bad practice, than to be prescriptive about what constitutes good practice. If the diagnostic basis for prescribing is often uncertain, the response of a rational healthcare system must be to reduce that uncertainty in pursuit of quality. We addressed the following three questions:

- Can we control for rational prescribing?
- Can we manage for rational prescribing?
- Can we educate for rational prescribing?

Can we control for rational prescribing?

Essentially, government has taken two approaches to controls. The first is the attempt to control the substances that can be prescribed to NHS patients. These controls begin with the creation of limited lists (largely blacklisted drugs of poor or absent efficacy or of unreasonable comparative cost). Over the years these lists have been extended and, as choice for doctor and patient becomes more limited, they have become more controversial.

The limiting of available drugs is taken a step nearer the preferences and habits of practising doctors by the creation of formularies, which is now widely encouraged. These may be created at practice level, at Family Health Service Authority (FHSA) level, or even at regional level. The Health Select Committee has suggested the creation of a "National Health Service prescribing list", which would eventually become a "national formulary".

At the practice level, the construction of a shared formulary has a powerful educational influence on the doctors concerned. When constructing the formulary, they are driven to review the relevant literature, to discuss therapeutic intentions, and to gain a large measure of co-ownership of the resulting list. There is a further benefit, if these formularies are seen to be indicative rather than prescriptive: departures from the formulary are not treated as misdemeanours but as the occasion for reviewing and discussing the reason.

As the field of application of formularies is extended from practice to district to region and so on, there are two consequences. Firstly, an increasing breadth and quality of expertise goes into the creation of the formulary. Secondly, the sense of the individual doctor's ownership of the formulary becomes increasingly dilute. None the less, there is an increasing trend towards shared and cooperative care between general practice and hospitals. Such shared care cannot be successful unless the hospital and general formularies are reconciled. The work of negotiating such shared formularies provides an important opportunity for multidisciplinary learning to take place, and acts as a model for continuing education relevant of the needs of specialists, GPs, and their patients.

If indeed, as seemed both likely and desirable by some members of our group, the NHS is presented with a "prescribing list", a number of interesting ethical and political considerations will arise. The creation of such limits to prescribing in the NHS would need to be widely discussed and publicised. It is essential that the clients of the service are told about any changes in their entitlements. It is not only healthcare professions who need ownership of a new formulary but also the patients. A major consequence of any limitation to the freedom to prescribe is that, although the overall aims of improved quality of care and distributive justice may be met, this will be at the cost, for some individuals, of some marginal benefits.

Let us imagine that, in a particular therapeutic class, drugs X and Y are preferred and included in the list. Drugs P, Q, and R are excluded, on the grounds of cost, and on the grounds that they convey no substantial therapeutic advantage over their cheaper competitors. It will always be true that for some patients drug P, Q, or R may achieve better results than either drug X or Y. Even if this is only a placebo response, this may be substantial for the individual, although only very marginal indeed in terms of the health service as a whole. Will the NHS GP be allowed to continue to prescribe drugs P, Q, and R, on the condition that the patient meets the full cost? This would certainly meet the goals of autonomy and beneficence for the individual patient, but at the cost of another key principle of the NHS—equity.

The second approach of the government to controlling prescribing is the attempt to limit spending. Indicative prescribing amounts have hitherto been based on FHSA historical data. There are already incentive schemes for GPs, who may receive £3000 for keeping within their target budgets. Sanctions for irrational prescribing might include fines or termination of contract.

The Health Select Committee wishes to see an extension of incentive schemes for all general practices, not only for fundholders, and also an extension of sanctions. However, it is interesting to note that these financial controls have not been considered independently of quality issues. The committee noted that under-prescribing, no less than over-prescribing, may indicate poor quality. They recommended that both incentives and sanctions "address quality of prescribing as well as quantity: it would be wrong if too great a pre-occupation with the cost issue in isolation were to encourage under-prescribing or have an adverse effect on patient care".

Clearly there is a danger if financial incentives and sanctions are insensitively applied. Without assessing clinical appropriateness, much will be lost from the quality of medical care. The basis of the relationship between doctor and patient is a fiduciary one: the patient must continue to trust the doctor to give him the best possible prescription, and he or she may be suspicious of a health service that rewards the doctor financially for withholding what the patient feels that he or she is entitled to receive.

Lastly, in order to put a brake on what some have described as the insatiable appetite of the human animal for the consumption of medication, government can impose prescription charges. At present in the UK only some 15% of prescriptions filled are subject to such charges—there are innumerable exemptions because of age, disease, unemployment, and so on. If these exemptions were reduced, or if some form of proportional co-payment was introduced, again the principle of equity in the health service would be seen to be damaged.

Can we manage for rational prescribing?

At our first meeting, the question was asked "Will the general practitioner in the future continue to be competent to prescribe?" Given the increasingly demanding desiderata for competent prescribing described earlier in this chapter, this question had to be taken seriously. It may well be that at the end of the 20th century the role of prescribing, traditionally the unique province of the doctor, should pass to others.

Already in very many general practices, the monitoring of patients with chronic disease has become the responsibility of the practice nurse. Most often this is supported by clinical guidelines and protocols. This means that it is the nurse who determines and recommends that the dose of, say, antihypertensive drugs, or insulin, or steroids should be varied. However, the GP still retains the responsibility and must formally endorse the alterations to treatment.

The change that we looked at, however, is much more radical than this. In future the sheer size and complexity of the prescribing task may cause us to think again about the unitary nature of the clinical transaction. We may need to disaggregate the clinical task. It might become the task of the GP, having explored the problem, to determine the therapeutic *strategy* but not to choose the specific drugs. The GP might specify what class of drugs are to be used, and in what sequence they should be prescribed. It would be the practice pharmacist's task to choose the particular drugs, to recommend the starting doses, to negotiate all this with the patient. This would entail not only a change in role but an important shift in responsibility. The monitoring of the patient's progress would then become a cooperative task between the practice nurse and the practice pharmacist. The GP's role would be to solve problems, and to consult in the on-going process.

Such a suggestion is likely to be greeted with deep distaste by the majority of GPs today. While the medical profession has become accustomed to rapid and radical changes in medical technology, the notion that these will entail rapid and radical changes in clinical roles, tasks, and responsibilities has not yet been widely acknowledged.

There are strong and convincing arguments against such team development. British general practice as an academic discipline has long endorsed the notion that the care of the patient is not a group process but rather is a personal relationship. How to conserve what is deeply valued (an intimate and continuing relationship between doctor and patient), while developing the breadth of experience, the freedom from isolation, and the added efficiency of teamwork, has become a major challenge. The challenge of rational prescribing now highlights this.

The benefits of such team work, and in particular a new cooperative relationship with pharmacists, are potentially very

The role of a primary care pharmacist

- Formulary management
- Medication review
- Prescription query
- Pharmacokinetic assessment
- Compliance assessment
- Drug counselling

great indeed—not only for the doctors and nurses in the practice but also for their patients. Primary care pharmacists (PCPs), based in practices, could become responsible for the pharmaceutical care of the practice population. They would also effect liaison with community and hospital pharmacists, would undertake domiciliary visits where necessary, and would certainly emerge as key players in the primary healthcare team of the future.

This model envisages not only a new type of pharmacist, but also a new type of GP. One of our group in support of this vision, quoted Marcel Proust: "The real art of discovery is not in finding new lands but seeing with new eyes."

Of course such changes in the structure and function of primary healthcare teams will probably begin in the larger and more entrepreneurial fundholding practices, some of which already employ community pharmacists to oversee repeat prescriptions and to manage the formulary. Analogous arrangements will then be necessary for small practices, and there will be major implications for the role and development of retail pharmacists, who make a unique and important contribution to health care in our system. This contribution must not be carelessly lost as an unintended consequence of other desired changes. It is possible to envisage experimentation with a number of new configurations between retail pharmacists and small practices. As with all such developments, if they are seen to respond to need and to be popular with patients, the diffusion will be wider and more rapid than we can now imagine.

We were aware of radical developments in the USA where the growth of managed health care has resulted in the development of so-called "managed pharmacy". There, pharmacy benefits management companies are now engaged in drug formulary development and management, disease management protocols, prescription processing, drug utilisation reviews, compliance management, and so on.

Developments in the USA are not necessarily or directly relevant to future developments in the NHS. But what is occurring in the USA, and the new role for practice pharmacists adumbrated in this chapter, amount to what organisation theorists would describe as a re-engineering of the therapeutic process. Should the therapeutic process be re-engineered in this way, there is little doubt that the fundamental principles and beliefs of British general practice would be seriously challenged. In particular there would be great anxieties that patients with established clinical conditions would become trapped in a bureaucratic and insensitive therapeutic machine, where clinical judgment would be overridden by protocols and where, instead of the therapy being fitted to the patient, the patient would be required to fit the treatment.

This real danger reinforces the need for GPs to develop further what have become their key skills. These include the simultaneous exercise of rational clinical problem solving and a sensitivity to implicit information and intuitive thinking. Far from diminishing the role of GPs by removing some of their traditional functions and replacing them with new ones, their role and effectiveness may be enhanced.

For the most compelling of scientific, economic, and organisational reasons, it is likely that the treatment of diseases in the future will be driven by elaborate protocols. The patient's condition may then be "understood" and "interpreted" not by the doctor exercising judgment, but by an increasingly powerful Bayesian analysis of biological data. The key role, then, for the GP, will be to subordinate the application of these theoretical protocols to the needs of the patient's unique human situation.

Can we educate for rational prescribing?

Limited lists, formularies, and budgets cannot in themselves achieve rational prescribing for the individual patient. In the very nature of things, control mechanisms tend to be rigid and unresponsive to unique situations and individuals. Consequently, rational prescribing requires not only control mechanisms that engender compliance but also educational activities that engender judgment.

The provenance of healthcare education, whether this is presented as new information, or as new skill training, colours the lessons that are learned. In chapter 1 the sources of information bias were discussed. A pharmaceutical company may appear to sponsor a course on the management of a disease but may be seen to promote one of its newer products. A specialist clinician may, similarly, be concerned with the promotion of his own and his hospital's services. The FHSA pharmaceutical advisor or medical director may be seen as policing cost, in the name of improving care. The importance of these insights is not to disenfranchise any of these (or other) contributors to education on prescribing, but rather to focus the learner's healthy scepticism.

General practitioners in England have for the past six years received prescription analyses and cost reports (PACT data); similar reports have been made available in Scotland, Wales, and Northern Ireland. The quality of these data have recently been markedly upgraded[11] so as to give GPs and practices up-to-date information about the levels and distribution of their prescribing. The volume and cost of prescribing is compared with local averages. Trends can be tracked, information on current national issues will now be included, and there will be links with the practice's own data. This impressive service, of course, will be directed mainly to those aspects of rationality in prescribing that have to do with costs: the link between the measures of volume and cost and other measures of quality (the level of case finding, the appropriateness and effectiveness of medication and so on) must be seen as implied rather than direct. In future, these latter markers of quality could be explicitly incorporated.

Medical and pharmaceutical advisors to FHSAs have been given pivotal roles in the attainment of better general practice prescribing. The role of these advisors, the nature of their activities, the opportunities and problems posed by their lines of accountability and professional solidarity are all ambiguous and complex. They can be seen simply as effecting a liaison between the practice and the authority. They can also be seen as ambassadors, counsellors, facilitators, coaches, instructors, or government inspectors.

Regional advisers in general practice and the (ambiguously) independent medical audit advisory groups (MAAGs) have an important part to play in providing a balanced educational programme in pursuit of rational prescribing. There is no reason why they cannot cooperate in this with other less disinterested players, provided the educational aims, methods, and evaluations are sound, and the personal, organisational, or commercial agendas are recognised and made explicit.

In particular, programmes should be jointly devised and presented by specialists in the relevant clincial fields, and experienced GP tutors who will be concerned to relate the perspectives of specialist medicine to the context of general practice. A benchmark for educational probity is that clinical controversy is robustly addressed.

The range of educational approaches that can be pursued to achieve rational prescribing is outwith the remit of this chapter. A number of principles are, however, worth rehearsing. In all adult learning, interactive work is more likely to result in subsequent behavioural change than is didactic instruction. If the educational material is drawn not only from theory but also from the doctor's own practice and records, the relevance of the education to the quality of the doctor's performance and the patient's care is made immediately apparent.

If the educational intention is to change not only the behaviour of the individual doctor, but of the whole primary healthcare team, multidisciplinary learning can address not only the question of rational prescribing but also the way in which the roles of doctors, nurses, pharmacists, receptionists, and patients interact.

In the UK over the past 20 years, small group learning has emerged as the most appropriate model for continuing medical education. Learning in small groups is powerfully reinforced, if the group is on-going, and if performance is repeatedly fed back to the group. In this way, medical audit becomes incorporated into medical education.

Conclusions

The achievement of rational prescribing will require major changes in the way in which we think about the whole clinical process. It will require change in the micro-organisation of health care at the practice and hospital level, and in the macro-organisation of the NHS. Traditional professional roles will be challenged, old tasks abandoned, and new ones acquired.

If there is one lesson that we have learned from the recent NHS changes, it is this. In addition to determining what changes we are aiming at, we have to negotiate a reasonable pace of change with those who must participate in it. Furthermore, a sensible and measured pace of change allows us to modify our original aims in the light of experience. Perhaps the achievement of rational prescribing could become such a model for rational development in the NHS.

References

1 The Audit Commission. *Prescription for improvement*. London: HMSO, 1994. (Health and Personal Social Services Report 1.)

2 Health select committee second report. *Priority setting in the NHS: the drug budget.* London: HMSO, 1994.

3 Riegger GA. Ace inhibitors in early stages of heart failure. *Circulation*, 1993; **87** (5 suppl IV): 117–9.

4 Einarson TR. Drug-related hospital admissions. *Ann Pharmacother* 1993; 27(7–8): 832–40.

5 Cormack J, Marinker M, Morrell D. *Practice: clinical management in general practice.* London: Kluwer Medical, 1987.

6 Crombie DL, Cross KW, Fleming DM. The problem with diagnostic variability in general practice. *J Epidemiol Community Health* 1992; 46, 447–54.

7 Jenkins R, Smeeton N, Shepherd M. *Classification of mental disorder in primary care.* Cambridge: Cambridge University Press, 1988. (Psychological Medicine. Monograph Supplement 12.)

8 Balint M. *The Doctor, his patient and the illness*. London: Tavistock Publications, 1964.

9 Marinker M. General practice and the new contract. In: *Greening The White Paper*. London: The Social Market Foundation, 1989: paper No. 4.

10 Balint M, Hunt J, Joyce D, Marinker M, Woodcott J. *Treatment or diagnosis*. London: Tavistock Publications, 1970.

11 Harris CM. Better feedback on prescribing for general practitioners. *BMJ* 1994; **309**: 309–356.

Chapter 7
How should changes in primary health care be evaluated?

Andrew Harris

Partner: MEDICAL ADVISERS SUPPORT CENTRE

Following Tomlinson, London seems set to be the social laboratory for experimental variations in the provision of primary health care. This will take place against the background of immense and possibly disruptive restructuring of the capital's hospital services. Most of the GP leadership (medicopolitical and academic) has expressed anxiety about the quality of services which will ensue. We asked our group to consider by what criteria they would judge the quality of the ensuing changes. Although London provides the example, the issues examined seem equally pertinent to any large UK conurbation.

Author:	Dr Andrew Harris	*Honorary Lecturer in General Practice, King's College, London; and primary care adviser*
Convenor:	Professor Marshall Marinker	
Members:	Dr Gene Fader	*Research Fellow, St Bartholomew's Hospital Medical School, University of London*
	Professor John Gabbay	*Director, Institute of Public Health Medicine, Wessex RHA*
	Dr Iona Heath	*General Practitioner, London*
	Mr John James	*Chief Executive, Kensington, Chelsea and Westminster Commissioning Agency*
	Dr Jonathan Shapiro	*Senior Fellow, Health Services Management Centre, Birmingham University*
	Dr David Sloan	*Director, Health Development, Redbridge and Waltham Forest DHA*
	Mr David Taylor	*Health Economist, The Audit Commission*
	Professor Alison While	*Department of Community Nursing, King's College London*

Introduction

London, like most other capital cities in the Western World, has proved to be a magnet for specialist services, teaching and research. Consequently inner London has for the last hundred years seen a relatively unchecked growth in the number and size of its specialist teaching hospitals. These service, teaching, and research facilities were created to serve a national, and not only a London need. However, throughout the second half of the century, again in common with other inner cities, there has been an exodus of population to the suburbs. In the UK, as the NHS has grown, the last 50 years has seen the widespread provision of healthcare facilities of similar quality to that in the capital, throughout the country. This shift of population out of inner conurbations, and the rapid development of excellent services nationwide, is the background to the growing belief that London was over-provided with hospital beds.

At the same time there was much evidence in inner London that primary health care was under resourced, compared with the rest of the country. Although there are many examples of excellent practices, there are also many worrying examples of serious under-performance. All these changes and perceptions formed the background to the Tomlinson enquiry. The Tomlinson report[1] recommended a correction of what was believed to be the over provision of hospital beds and the under provision of good health care in the community.

The Government's response was *Making London better*.[2] A key recommendation was the proposal to build up primary care resources, so as to provide a much better quality of care, not least in order to offset the proposed reduction in hospital based facilities. A central assumption of both Tomlinson and the Government's response, was that the quality of health care in London would be greatly enhanced, and the cost contained, by creating a significant shift of resources from secondary to primary care. We were asked to address the question "How should we evaluate the expected changes?" This chapter, influenced by those discussions, deals with the issues raised, the problems encountered, and the suggestions offered.

What are London's health care challenges?

The most pressing reason for establishing the Tomlinson enquiry was the escalating demands from the acute sector for capital redevelopment. Although London is unique in many respects, the pattern of inner city social needs, the relative underdevelopment of primary health care, and the pressure of the market to rationalise the hospital sector, are familiar in other inner cities across the developed world.

London's healthcare problems are summarised in the King's Fund commission report.[3] A subsequent King's Fund paper emphasised the social and long term healthcare needs of older people.[4] Following the Tomlinson report, Maxwell[5] identified the problems facing London, and pointed out that other cities shared the same problems. Jarman[6, 7] has criticised Tomlinson's assertion that London is over-bedded. Judge, examining data from the 1991 census and NHS statistics, suggested that inner city London had significantly greater healthcare needs than outer London. In some respects they were greater than those of other conurbations in England.[8] The basis of the Tomlinson assumptions is therefore seriously challenged.

The conclusions of Maxwell and Judge are summarised below.

Special problems affecting health care in London

- Exceptional poverty and deprivation alongside affluence
- A shortage of affordable housing of reasonable quality
- A multi-ethnic population
- Relatively weak primary and community based health and social services
- A relative deficiency in the provision of nursing homes and residential care for the elderly
- A high proportion of people living alone
- An exceptional degree of population mobility
- A heavy reliance on accident and emergency departments and short admissions to acute hospitals
- An over-provision but fragmentation of specialist facilities
- Inadequate funding for the large number of hospitals

It should be borne in mind, however, that what is unique to London is not the categories but the size of the problems.

London is particularly characterised by areas of high unemployment, overcrowding in many districts, a large daytime commuter and tourist population, and a fourfold concentration of ethnic minorities compared with the rest of the UK.

The present state of play

The government earmarked a substantial resource in order to implement *Making London better*. The mechanisms of implementation are complex and can often confuse. The areas covered by inner city family health service authorities (FHSAs) are now designated as London implementation zones (LIZs). While FHSAs and other statutory authorities continue to exercise their commissioning functions, a London implementation group (LIG) was established to enable these commissioning authorities and other agencies to implement the proposals of the LIZs. In addition, the LIG has also commissioned a number of projects from voluntary agencies. A large number and variety of projects are now underway and are being planned.

From an examination of statements and plans emerging from the LIG, we have attempted to categorise these projects under three headings. The position is of course dynamic; the information given in Table I captures projects underway at the time of writing. It suggests the range and variety of activities: this gives some suggestion of the complexity of the task of evaluation.

Prerequisites for evaluation

Before a useful framework for future evaluation can be constructed, four prerequisites can be identified. These are:

- An adequate baseline of data: if change is to be measured, we need to know the starting position
- Clear statements of intention at three levels: we are interested in the intentions of the strategy for London; we are interested in the implementation of the policy; we want to know what were the expected impacts on the health care of people and populations

115

TABLE I Summary of London implementation zone (LIZ) plans.*†

	Getting the basics right	Innovation	Primary/secondary care interface
Premises	GP surgeries Community health clinics	Extended primary care centres Community houses/day centres	Polyclinics Rehabilitation Intermediate care beds GP beds
Out of hours	Telephone advice GP locum cover	GP cooperatives On-call nurses	GPs in A & E Primary care minor injuries centres
Staffing	Practice staff CHS staff Community consultant Mental health services	Extended PHCT Nurse practitioners Extended roles for pharmacists Mobile dentistry Pathology testing	GP outreach clinics Discharge and referral systems Substitution projects "Hospital at home"
Information techonology/communications	GP computerisation Validating practice lists CHS information	FHSA links—fax, directories	Information strategies
Training and professional development	PHCT training, team work, CME Primary care development Business support Dentistry skills	Multidisciplinary training Clinical audit, local mentors, postgraduate centres, lectureships, diplomas, nurse specialist needs	Nurse retraining Conversion courses

TABLE I *Continued*

	Getting the basics right	Innovation	Primary/secondary care interface
Inter-agency commissioning and consumer affairs	Purchaser development Needs assessment Locality projects Health strategies Local authority liaison Communications Professional advisers Consumer services	Special needs: ethnic minority homelessness, drug and alcohol abuse Community care Health education Patient advocacy/participation Benefits advice Social workers Quality standards	Carer support Elderly "sitting" Outreach respite care
Research	Evaluation of programme Monitoring	Community projects	Interface projects RCT domiciliary stroke Bed audit, day care study A & E costs evaluation

* Based on data kindly supplied by LIG.
† CME = continuing medical education, CHS = community health services, FHSA = family health service authority, PHCT = primary health care team, RCT = randomised controlled trial.

- Specific criteria: we believe that these intentions should be expressed in unambiguous terms, so that we would have criteria by which to judge the changes
- Early warning of success/failure: in order to avoid a waste of resources in pointless evaluation, we believe that every project should have explicitly stated failure criteria; it would be wasteful to pursue the evaluation of an initiative which was clearly failing by a wide margin.

Frameworks

We were divided on the subject of what to evaluate. There was a purist argument that only health outcomes should be measured. The current jargon is "health gain". A more pragmatic view prevailed, however. There are proxies for outcomes which could be measured. Elements of the processes of health care would give strong indication about whether the health service was functioning healthily. Following this discussion we began to construct a framework, which we now offer for consideration. We suggest that *Making London better* can be evaluated at three levels:

- *The strategy:* we wish to evaluate the overall goals and intentions of the policy. Is the strategy "competent"?
- *The implementation:* we believe it important to evaluate the way in which the strategy had been translated into more detailed policies, plans, and projects
- *The impact:* what are the effects of the changes on all those involved? What are the impacts on health, care, and on the function and morale of the healthcare workers involved?

At each of these three levels, we wish to ask three questions, so that the evaluation would be precisely located, permitting us to choose a variety of marker topics. These questions are:

- What is to be achieved?
- By which criteria will the results be judged?
- What methods should be used to evaluate?

What follows is an examination of the framework at all three levels.

The strategy

We began by asking "Has there been a clear and visionary strategic intention in *Making London better*?" There are five characteristics by which to judge strategic competence.

Principles

We believe that *Making London better* should be judged in relation to Maxwell's six dimensions of quality. However, we recognise that principles are expressed at a very general level, and therefore they may mean different things to different actors in the healthcare arena. Not only might each actor understand the terms differently, but the terms might well be prioritised in a different way.

We looked at a model composed of three major stakeholders: government, providers and consumers. The origins of this model are described in chapter 1. To examine it, we devised a game that consisted of ranking the Maxwell's six dimensions of quality[9] as they might be expressed by, for example, a health minister, the medical director of a trust, and a patient. Maxwell himself (personal communication) suggested that the six principles were to be used not as guidelines for implementation, but rather as guidelines for evaluation. He did not in any sense wish to suggest a hierarchy of values. If a particular service did not score well in terms of accessibility or efficiency, this was the area that had to be addressed and redressed. None the less, we believe that these six dimensions could be used as a template for judging whether the strategy achieved its objectives.

Maxwell's six dimensions of quality

- Access to services
- Relevance to need
- Effectiveness
- Equity
- Social acceptability
- Efficiency

Time

Strategy should be long term, concerned with looking at benchmarks year on year, and sensitive to the need to pace change. There was considerable discussion about the evidence for long term thinking in *Making London better*. Had some sort of timetable been suggested, had the pace and power of change been related to such matters as the availability of resources, conflicts between objectives of stakeholders[10, 11] and the ability of healthcare personnel to adapt to some quite far reaching changes in their roles and tasks, it might be possible to evaluate the competence of this programme. However, one view is that it is unrealistic to expect a detailed timetable, and indeed, that the presence of such a timetable might damage the process. At all events, long term plans need to be constantly revised, in order to take on board the inevitable changes in circumstances that are to be expected but cannot be predicted in detail.

Comprehensiveness

How comprehensive is the strategic approach of *Making London better*? Research has shown clear links between housing, education, employment, social status, and the health of Londoners.[12, 13] However, there is little evidence that those responsible in London for housing, education, employment, and so on are involved in the implementation of the strategy or indeed in the district development plans for primary care. Jacobson[14] notes the absence of a clear public health function which would link local purchasing plans to the health needs of Londoners.

Coherence

The list of topics given in the examples of LIZ projects earlier, under each of which projects are envisaged, certainly suggests a wide scatter of concerns. It is however very difficult to make any judgment about the comprehensive nature of these, without relating them in some way to an over-arching design. Yet such a design can only be based on an estimation of the healthcare needs to which reponses are required. The view held by some, that *Making London better* suggests a top-down view of management, is a valid one. However, what can appear to be an *ad hoc* and untidy list of activities, may, on examination, be found to be a sensitive reponse to challenges that are locally perceived. The fact

Five characteristics for judging strategic competence

- *Principles:* what principles underlie the strategy and its evaluations?
- *Timescale:* is the strategy long term?
- *Comprehensiveness:* are housing, education, employment, etc, linked with implementation of the strategy?
- *Coherence:* has cooperative planning between different sorts of authority, including medical education, been incorporated?
- *Revision:* are there provisions for revisions of strategy?

that they are not evidently part of a grand public health plan may not be as damning a criticism of rational policy as it might at first appear.

A coherent strategy would reveal signs that different aspects of health and social care were interacting. Concepts can be neatly categorised, but the problems of an individual patient, or of a local community, will always be found to be multi-dimensional. They will include particular morbidities, social circumstances, environmental problems, and so on. Since health is not simply a biological but also a social concept, a strategic plan for London should include the possibility of cooperative planning and sharing of projects between different sorts of authorities—those concerned with primary health care, housing, and education, for example. Bosanquet and Leese[15] have shown that practices in socially deprived areas are less able to respond to development incentives than those in more affluent areas. A strategic plan that aims to be coherent would therefore include the monitoring of resource allocation to detect whether the Tomlinson investment is in fact reversing what Julian Tudor Hart[16] called the inverse care law.

Rees and Wass[17] suggested out that the effort demanded for reorganising the hospital service along the lines suggested by Tomlinson will leave very little energy for innovation in undergraduate education. Reeve[18] has argued that research institutions will be damaged by competition in an internal market and has called for secure mechanisms for funding the

121

cost of clinical research. Swales[19] has stressed that teaching cannot be divorced from patient care and that, like research, teaching needs special support and protection in terms of staff, time, and money. All these observations, concerned primarily with the needs of teaching hospitals, are no less relevant in developing teaching and research in primary care—the focus of the Tomlinson initiative. The conference on educational implications of Tomlinson for general practice[20] voiced other concerns—about flexibility of career paths, the continued dominance of the pharmaceutical industry in continuing education, and the absence of a secure mechanism for dealing with the under-performing GP. Would a coherent strategy show evidence of response to all these concerns?

Revision

Provision should be made for constant revision of the detailed intentions and the adequacy of performance. Five year plans are best thought of as five year plans reviewed annually. Are there provisions for this in *Making London better*?

Implementation

Strategy is converted into reality by the processes of implementation. This converts the strategic intention into specific objectives with defined timescales, objectives, lines of accountability, and so on.

It could be argued that if the strategic plan meets the sort of criteria suggested above, and if the impact of the projects generated by *Making London better* is positive, there is no need for evaluators to be concerned with the mechanisms that brought about the results. However, some of our group feel that there are a number of good reasons for looking at the processes—the ways in which the implementation is conceived and functions. Implementation could therefore be looked at in terms of the clarity of its objectives; the sense of ownership created among those involved in the implementation; the simplification and shortening of lines of accountability; the devolution of responsibility to those close to the provision of the service; a sensitivity to the need for cooperative work, the implementation of policies in partnership with a variety of different agencies caring for the same areas of social and healthcare concerns.

Two examples will suffice. In Sheffield[21] a group of practices cooperated in an exercise aimed at evaluating their current services and developing their primary care teams. They were able to do this because they had defined their objectives and standardised the way in which they prepared their data about morbidity, attendance rates, referral, prescribing, and so on. What is admirable about this project, is the degree to which all those concerned were able to share ownership of the idea.

A second example is reported by Benson and Miller.[22] Here again, ownership was the key. A technique for the development of standards was developed, which gave due weight to the views of consumers and of the "less articulate providers". What resulted was a set of standards that covered such aspects as continuity of care, the reduction of risk to patients, patient compliance and satisfaction, aspects of accessibility, cost, and much else.

Impacts

We use the term "impacts" to refer to the results of policies, the ways in which the policies change and improve the care that patients receive. We chose to use the word "impacts" rather than "outcomes" in order to go beyond outcomes in a strictly Donabedian sense—that is, measures of actual health gain by individuals or populations. Sometimes it is appropriate, adequate, or simply necessary to measure proxies for these outcomes, and these are included in the term "impacts".

Impacts can be judged in relation to a number of evaluative models. Maxwell's six dimensions was one such that we have examined. The redistribution of resources between different parts of London, the recognition of differences in healthcare need and social deprivation between different neighbourhoods, would signal achievement of equity. The development of new services for patients currently deemed to be less than well served by the current services would signal the achievement of greater relevance and equity.

The Royal College of General Practitioners developed a series of indicators of good practice, published under the title *What sort of Doctor?*[23] This technique, at once educational and evaluative,

might well be used at intervals over the next few years to monitor changes in clinical competence, appropriateness of the service, staff morale, and much else. Patient satisfaction measures have long been held to be reliable in terms of the social acceptability of the service, but unreliable in terms of its clinical effectiveness and efficiency. Vuori[24] and Baker,[25] however, have shown the validity of patient satisfaction measures as measures of quality of care.

The classical model of medical audit, measuring structures, processes and outcomes, is associated with the name of Avedis Donabedian. This provides us with one of the most powerful models for evaluation. Changes in the structure of care, although they do not directly measure changes in the provision of health care, let alone improvements in health, are none the less important prerequisites of such change.

Some 75% of the initial investment in *Making London better* has gone towards projects classified as "Getting the basics right". To a large extent these are elements of structure: the provision of surgery premises and community health clinics; the provision of good locum cover and telephone advice services; the development of staff; community health services; the provision of community consultants and staff in the mental health service; the provision of information technology; and the development of training and management support. All of these can be seen as part of "structure", but with a clear relationship to the delivery of effective and efficient care. They are, within our definition, also "impacts".

In "Getting the basics right" there is an overlap between processes and outcomes. Many processes can be seen to be intermediate or proxy outcomes. Examples would include the good functioning of primary healthcare teams and the quality of medical records. Other important proxy measures are the attainment of the prescribed targets in the GP contact. Another example might be the measurement of average consultation times in general practice: Howie *et al*[26] has demonstrated that longer consultations result in more appropriate communication between doctor and patient.

One of our group, a London GP has recently found herself spending up to two hours on the telephone, seeking the appropriate emergency admission of an eldery patient to a medical unit. The problem of arranging hospital admissions for acutely ill patients in London has been well documented.[27] How would the measurement of "admission time" shorten over the coming five years? How soon would these improvements be seen?

Perhaps the most intriguing suggestion to arise in our discussion is that some cohort of patients might be identified to represent different ages, medical conditions and social situations. The examples we would choose are the mentally ill and homeless, Asian adults with type II diabetes, children with asthma, and young drug abusers. Developing clear criteria about the structure process and outcome elements that should improve over time, these cohorts of patients could be tracked and their care monitored.

Methods

Given the fact that there are constant changes in healthcare problems, social circumstances, the economy, and so on, there is very considerable difficulty in linking cause to effect. There may be changes for the better or for worse in primary care, but we would wish to be able to ascribe these to the intentions and processes of the Tomlinson implementation.

We have been much concerned with the question "How much evaluation?" All evaluations entail the use of resources. There has to be, therefore, a trade-off between those resources devoted to providing the health service, and those devoted to evaluation—to assuring that the service remains true to its intentions and to the needs of its consumers. Therefore the notion that all projects can and should be rigorously evaluated is not sustainable. There has to be a sensitive and sensible choice of what to evaluate. On what basis should this choice be made?

Maxwell had suggested that his six dimensions of quality be used as yardsticks to determine which dimensions are deficient or absent. Those projects initiated under the aegis of *Making London better* which are designed to redress serious shortfalls in these dimensions might well receive priority when it comes to choosing what to evaluate. New services designed for the homeless and the mentally ill are obvious examples.

Most research, not least research in primary medical care, is distorted by the understandable wish to measure the measurable. The fact that some aspect of the provision of health care or some aspect of health care outcome is easily defined and measured does not of itself constitute an argument for giving this priority. We

125

should be concerned to quantify, or if necessary to make a qualitative assessment of those aspects of health care which are important to people—which respond to evident need.

A major problem in measuring change is the validity and reliability of the baseline or starting measurement. However, because of differences between localities—differences in social structure and resources—the "playing field" between different localities is rarely level. The absence of adequate baselines for most health policy implementation has led to the view that cost comparisons can rarely be used to measure relative efficiency.[28] The measurement of change, therefore must relate to the specific antecedent situation. The evaluation must be specific to both place and time. Failure to observe these elementary requirements can lead to dangerously misleading conclusions.

We recognised that comparisons between different institutions or localities are fraught with the possibility of error. The social context of the health service is as imporant as its content, when judgments are being made about the impact of changes on quality. Comparison with past performance may be a much more secure indication of the effects of *Making London better*. Best of all, evaluations should be made against clearly defined benchmarks which reflect a consensus about quality. The problems in reaching such consensus are discussed in chapter 1.

Finally, there is a real conflict between the need to create as wide an ownership as possible of the processes of evaluation, on the one hand, and the need for expertise, on the other. The wider the involvement of healthcare personnel in evaluation, the more likely they are to become committed to the goals of quality that the evaluation is intended to support. The greater the concentration of evaluation in the hands of experts and professional institutions, the more confidence we can place in the results. Ways must be found of trying to accomplish both desirable ends—perhaps the widespread involvement of individuals and agencies in the collection of evidence leaving the control of the research in the hands of experts.

Conclusions

In examining the question "How should we evaluate change", we have been impressed by the complexity of the task. It is not always easy to find consensus, as is exemplified by the fact that the following conclusions are not unanimously shared by the present authors. The most salient are:

- We have reservations about the strategic competence of *Making London better*, and are therefore uncertain that it will be possible to mount a strategic evaluation. Although it might be possible to carry out a number of piecemeal evaluations, a framework should be established such that a consideration of the sum of all the evaluations attempted will allow an overall judgment to be made
- The criteria chosen, and the evaluations carried out, should show a sensitivity to people and their experiences, and focus on areas of conflict between objectives of stakeholders rather than a slavish adherence to theory and concepts
- Ownership of the changes should be as wide as possible, in order to ensure that where a consensus is arrived at, it is based as securely as possible on the values of the citizens and professionals concerned, so that their implementation is enabled.
- The very act of determining criteria, the exploration of how they may be measured, should in themselves create that "reflection in action", which Schön[29] describes as the cardinal virtue of professionalism. If this can be brought about, it may be the most important and pervasive benefit of the Tomlinson enquiry and the government's response.

References

1 The Tomlinson Report. *Report of the inquiry into London's health service, medical education and research.* London: HMSO, 1993.
2 Department of Health. *Making London better.* London: Department of Health, 1993.
3 King's Fund Commission on the Future of London's Acute Health Services. *London health care 2010, changing the future service in the capital.* London: King's Fund Institute, 1992.
4 Boyle S, Sinaje C. *Primary health care in London. Quantifying the challenge.* London: King's Fund Institute, 1993.
5 Maxwell R. Other cities, same problems. In: *London after Tomlinson. Reorganizing big city medicine.* London: BMJ, 1993.
6 Jarman B. Is London over-bedded? *BMJ* 1993; **306**: 979–82.
7 Jarman B. *The crisis in London medicine: how many beds does the capital need?* London: University of London, 1994.
8 *London: key facts.* London: King's Fund Institute, 1992.
9 Maxwell RJ. Dimensions of quality revisited: from thought to action. *Quality in Health Care* 1992; **1**: 171–7.
10 GMSC. Response to Tomlinson Report. *BMJ* 1992; **305**: 1369.

11 Response of Greater London Association of Community Health Councils to the Inquiry into London's health service, medical education and research. 1992.

12 Blaxter M. *Health and lifestyles*. London: Tavistock Routledge, 1990.

13 Benzeval M, Judge K, Soloman M. *The health status of Londoners: a comparative perspective*. London: King's Fund, 1992. (London Initiative Working Paper No 1.)

14 Jacobson B. Public health in inner London. *BMJ* 1992; **305**: 1344–7.

15 Bosanquet N, Leese B. Family doctors and innovation in general practice. *BMJ* 1988; **296**: 1576–80.

16 Tudor Hart J. The inverse care law. *Lancet* 1971; **1**: 405–12.

17 Rees L, Wass J. Undergraduate medical education. *BMJ* 1993; **306**: 258–61.

18 Green M. Clinical research. In: *London after Tomlinson*. BMJ Publishing Group, 1993: 63–76.

19 Swales JD. Postgraduate medical education. In: *London after Tomlinson. Reorganizing big city medicine*. Publishing Group, London: BMJ 1993: 88–93.

20 Educational implications of Tomlinson for general practice. In: *Proceedings of Tomlinson task force conference, 31 Jan 1994*. London.

21 Improving quality through interpractice collaboration. *Quality in primary health care. A report of forum on quality in health care*. London: Royal Society of Medicine, 1993.

22 Benson D, Miller J. *An ambulatory quality assurance and quality management system*. Indianapolis: Methodist Hospital of Indiana, 1989.

23 *What sort of doctor?* London: Royal College of General Practitioners, 1985. (Report No 23).

24 Vuori H. Patient satisfaction: an attribute or an indicator of quality care. *J Health Care Quality Assurance* 1988; **1**(2): 29–32.

25 Baker R, Whitfield M. Measuring patient satisfaction: a test of construct validity. *Quality Health Care* 1992; **1**: 104–9.

26 Howie JGR, Parker AMD, Heaney DJ, Hepton JL. Long to short consultation ratio: a proxy measure of quality in general practice. *Br J Gen Pract* 1991; **4**: 48–52.

27 Jenkins C, Bartholomew J, Gelder F, Morrell D. Arranging hospital admissions for acutely ill patients. *Br J Gen Pract* 1994; **44**: 251–4.

28 Bartlett, Le Grand J. In: Robinson R, Le Grand J, editors. *Evaluating the NHS reforms*. London: King's Fund Institute.

29 Schön DA. *The reflective practitioner*. New York: Basic Books, 1983.

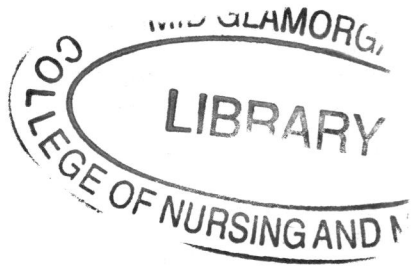

Index

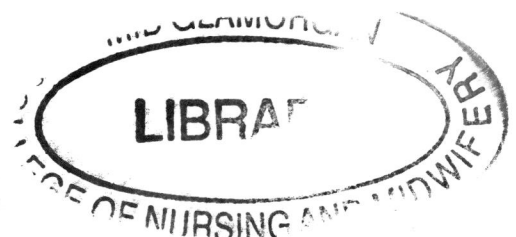